THE CARNIVORE'S
MANIFESTO

...IRE'S
MAN!FESTO

EATING WELL,
EATING RESPONSIBLY,
AND
EATING MEAT

PATRICK MARTINS

WITH MIKE EDISON

Foreword by Alice Waters

Drawings by Anne Saxelby

LITTLE, BROWN AND COMPANY
NEW YORK   BOSTON   LONDON

Little, Brown and Company
Hachette Book Group
237 Park Avenue, New York, NY 10017
littlebrown.com

First Edition: June 2014

Little, Brown and Company is a division of Hachette Book Group, Inc. The Little, Brown name and logo are trademarks of Hachette Book Group, Inc.

The publisher is not responsible for websites (or their content) that are not owned by the publisher.

The Hachette Speakers Bureau provides a wide range of authors for speaking events. To find out more, go to hachettespeakersbureau.com or call (866) 376-6591.

ISBN 978-0-316-25624-7

LCCN 2014937387

10 9 8 7 6 5 4 3 2 1

RRD-C

Printed in the United States of America

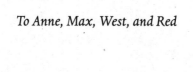

To Anne, Max, West, and Red

Contents

Contents

Foreword

Alice Waters

There are many ways to engage people about the crisis of this planet: I attempt to feed people ideas. Michael Pollan tells amazing stories. Eric Schlosser is a muckraking journalist of the first order. Vandana Shiva is a passionate orator. With each perspective, we add a necessary layer of complexity and depth to the food movement—and with this important new book, Patrick Martins brings a provocative and original voice to the discourse on food systems and sustainability.

At first, Patrick's humor and outrageous proclamations make you feel that he might just be making it all up. But there are deep wisdom and common sense in every chapter. An overarching theme emerges loudly and clearly— that we need to change our ways. Influenced by his mentor Carlo Petrini, president and founder of Slow Food International, Patrick is bold and willing to say what he feels and what he thinks, no matter how irreverent or shocking it might be. This is the message he compellingly delivers: If we eat and buy with intention, and focus on the pleasures of the table, our lives will be changed. (This is the Slow Food message—no surprise, as Patrick was the founding president of Slow Food USA.) Patrick's hilarious and exuberant rant shows us how easy and practical it is to do this. This is not a book about denying oneself—by deftly incorporating his knowledge of music, literature, and art into his writing, Patrick seduces us into finding pleasure in the righteous places.

THE CARNIVORE'S
MANIFESTO

The Revolution Starts Now

This book is an action-based approach to eating meat and living well on the planet Earth. It is about pleasure, and dignity, and fairness.

Every year Americans eat more than ten billion livestock. Unfortunately, most of these animals are the product of inhumane, nonsustainable, and cruel factory farming, the stuff of fast food and supermarket specials. It's a system that is bad for animals, is bad for people, and punishes an overtaxed environment.

THE CARNIVORE'S MANIFESTO effects a path to liberating ourselves from fast food and corporate agriculture and the destruction they bring. THE CARNIVORE'S MANIFESTO recognizes that a virtuous alternate American farm system has always existed, and has incredible potential to grow as a viable option to feed all Americans.

When it comes to the sort of greedy corporate farming and aberrant agriculture that supplies most Americans with their meat, we are completely in solidarity with our vegetarian friends. It is our belief that no one should be subjected to the unacceptable and harsh practices of that system.

The meat we celebrate is the righteous kind, from healthy animals of sound genetics that have been treated humanely and allowed to pursue their natural instincts. Antibiotics and growth hormones are not part of the system. The environment is respected, and fair labor is practiced.

Unfortunately, not everyone has access to quality food all the time, but all people deserve to eat this way. We dismiss the claim that good food is elitist, and that we should accept low standards of food quality for anyone. We applaud anything that moves the dial in the right direction, away from the Industrial Food Complex that has betrayed our trust: slowing down, eating meat in season, investing in local businesses, or getting cozy with your butcher.

This is a practical guide. We aren't confusing day-to-day life with impossible-to-achieve ideals, nor do we think we can create some sort of feel-good food utopia—the B in pretty much every BLT in the nation comes from a cruel system—but we are certain we should strive for it.

Following the advice in this book will ensure that you have a better relationship with the world around you and the food on your plate. You will feel better and have more fun.

Welcome to THE CARNIVORE'S MANIFESTO.

It boggles the mind when food is confused with fashion. Food is not a handbag; it is about sustenance and survival. It is the ultimate intimacy — you put it in your mouth. You put it in your body.

There is no bigger issue of our time than our food supply and the earth's ability to provide it for us. On every front, we are spoiling our nest. The thin layer of topsoil that feeds the planet is fraying like a cheap suit. Global warming is turning agricultural havens into deserts. Pesticides are poisoning a water supply that is quickly drying up in many areas. Our livestock are so overbred for fast growth that their bones are weak — a quarter of all chickens arrive at the slaughterhouse already injured and in pain. Antibiotics are fed to animals because they are presumed to be too sick to live without them, and humans who eat them, especially children, are becoming immune to certain medicines because of this chemically tainted food chain. We have lost most of the independent farms in this country. We need action!

My company, Heritage Foods USA, moves sixty thousand pounds of pasture-raised heritage and rare-breed pork and beef every week, and five times that amount of meat in October, November, and December because of all the turkeys, geese, and goats that are naturally ready for harvest during the holidays. Working with some of our nation's best farmers and chefs to get this food on the table is an honor, a responsibility, and a privilege that we cherish.

The reason we focus on pure heritage and rare-breed animals—like Red Wattle pigs and Narragansett turkeys—as opposed to their overbred commodity counterparts—is that many of these less common breeds have been pushed to the brink of extinction because they don't grow fast enough or produce enough lean meat to satisfy the corporate demand for maximum profit. A corporate chicken, the kind favored by fast-food companies, is hardly a chicken at all. It is a hot genetic mess of an animal.

There are dozens of varieties of cows, pigs, sheep, goats, chickens, ducks, geese, and turkeys. Each type looks different, acts different, tastes different, and comes from a different agricultural tradition, but from the perspective of the boardroom, there is little incentive to raise these beasts, even though many of them are renowned for their taste.

Maintaining rare and heritage breeds is crucial for a healthy and safe food supply. The viability of the livestock population depends on a strong genetic base. Novel pathogens, natural or man-made, can wipe out one variety while having no effect on another, which means that relying on only one or two is dangerous—we have to keep rare and heritage breeds viable by creating an active market for them.

Heritage Foods USA is responsible for moving whole animals, nose to tail. Selling every piece is the key to sustainability and to supporting the farmers who supply us, but it's a real challenge to sell all the parts from all the pigs and cattle that come in all year round. Thankfully, a network of visionary restaurants and a constellation of home chefs around the country are committed to ordering consistently and often.

My first run at the meat business was selling heritage turkeys, and for that I have to thank Frank Reese, the owner of the most important poultry farm in America. His farm in Kansas is a seething cauldron of biodiversity—he has dozens of poultry breeds, and in many cases his is the last farm in the world to be home to these breeds. Let me tell you how I found myself out there with his birds, listening to him talk so passionately about the need for more Americans to consume sustainable, heritage poultry.

In the spring of 1998 I had the cosmically great fortune of being in the right place at the right time, at a dinner at Remi in New York, where Slow Food founder Carlo Petrini happened to be dining. As usual, he was captivating the entire room, gesticulating like a wild man while preaching the virtues of sustainability in his Piedmontese dialect, keeping everyone laughing, but also delivering an unassailable gut check when it came to the realities of his cause. The owner, Francesco Antonucci, did me the great favor of introducing me to Carlo, and I quickly became a rapt disciple of Slow Food.

Carlo began Slow Food in 1986, largely to counter the homogenizing effects of fast food and its invasion of the Old World. Slow Food's first act was brutal in its simplicity, its message bell-clear to Italians: When the first McDonald's opened on the Spanish Steps of Rome, Carlo and his crew of high-minded anarchists from Bra, Italy, sat there and ate pasta in protest. Slow Food. It is now an international nonprofit movement dedicated to promoting producers, ingredients, regional cuisines, and biodiversity in the food supply.

Soon after our chance meeting at Remi, Carlo invited me to come to Italy to work with him. By then the Slow Food movement had about thirty thousand members, mostly in Europe. I arrived just months before Slow Food put on its second Salone del Gusto in Turin. Every single person of Carlo's hundred-person staff was working every waking moment to turn this event—which took over the entire Lingotto Fiat factory in Turin—into something of a miracle.

The Salone was an amusement park for food lovers— almost every artisanal food in the world was represented there, and you could taste them all in the Grand Market Hall or in classroom-style educational seminars led by experts. One hundred thousand people attended the Salone— no one had expected half that—and the publicity it generated helped Slow Food transition from an Italian organization to a global one. The year after the Salone, Slow Food membership swelled to over sixty thousand in sixty countries.

As Carlo became more of an international figure, he refined his message, although he never toned down his delivery. He is an amazing speaker, as anyone who has ever heard him in action can testify, the kind of guy who can talk his way into or out of anything, whether it is dodging a speeding ticket or igniting a movement.

The only truly modern answer to the question of how to deal with food, he repeatedly said, is *eco-gastronomy*, an understanding of what quality food is but also the knowledge of where it comes from. Being a gastronome alone, he continued, was gluttonous, and the people who only celebrated food on their plate were plainly stupid. On the other hand, ecologists and environmentalists were largely born of do-gooding American eggheads, and they were suicidally boring. Taste combined with traceability was the only answer—the unified theory, as physicists might say—and Carlo steered his movement to educate the public about good, clean, and fair food. At the same time, he never forgot to have fun.

The crucial Slow Food project that put the *eco* into practice was the virtual Slow Food Ark of Taste. Onto this imaginary but much-vaunted Ark, Slow Food boarded endangered foods with the goal of promoting them—the kind that have been pushed to the brink of extinction because of apathy or a corporate food culture that only respects a fast-faster-fastest mentality and profits at any cost. The international Ark grew to be a true catalog of biodiversity and was the perfect metaphor to bring to a country steeped in Old Testament lore.

Carlo loved the idea of his movement getting a foothold in America, the country responsible for starting the plague of fast food that was now infecting the world. Fueled by the success of the Salone, Carlo and I took two three-week marathon tours of the United States. We stopped in more than a dozen cities and talked to foodies before there even was such a word, and we were blown away by the depth of America's true gastronomic tradition, especially when it came to beer, wine, cheese, and bread. The amazing people we met on farms, in restaurants, and in homes were the leaders of the new food movement.

When we returned to Italy, I worked to capitalize on our goodwill tours and raise Slow Food membership in the States, so that we might have the funds to start a national headquarters in New York. I spent my days clanging away at my typewriter, firing off press releases and updates on Carlo's activities and our office happenings, and announcing the opening of new chapters.

Stories sprang up like poppies—we seemed to be in every major newspaper and magazine in the country. Suddenly we were receiving dozens of e-mails and calls to our toll-free number from people interested in paying $60 to become a member and receive the Slow Food magazine, which was appropriately called *Slow*. Once we had a few members signed up in a given city or town, I would pester them to hold a meeting of local members with the goal of starting a local chapter, or *convivium*, as we called it at the time. These were great folks, some of the most inspiring activists I have ever met. By March of 2000 I had achieved Carlo's first goal of 2,000 memberships in the States and was sent home with my Italian coconspirator, Serena Di Liberto, to run Slow Food USA out of my apartment in New York.

When I arrived back home, I realized that our successful

fund-raising and ambition had only created a greater need to raise money, to pay for the expense of a real office and a staff, which were needed to support the infrastructure of a growing movement. What we needed was a singular project that would galvanize and focus the current membership and convert others to the cause, all while also keeping Slow Food in the news. And thus the Ark became the vehicle—while signing up members, organizing events, and publishing our national newsletter, the *Snail,* I was busy getting biblical, boarding agricultural products onto our American Ark.

We boarded many foods, like rare varieties of apricots and apples, but the heritage turkey was by far our ideal poster child: It was American, everyone ate it, it even had its own holiday. The traditional, tastier breeds of turkey had been pushed aside in favor of larger-breasted and faster-growing birds concocted in corporate laboratories. For breeds like Bourbon Red, Narragansett, and Jersey Buff, only a few dozen breeding birds were alive and in action. We needed to do something—and fast—or these testaments to deliciousness would go the way of the dodo.

In 2001 we sent out the press release announcing the heritage turkey breeds' ceremonial entry onto the Ark of Taste, and soon Marian Burros wrote a *New York Times* article announcing that the following year Slow Food USA would begin selling these rare birds to Slow Food members. We were surprised—we weren't quite ready to get into the retail meat business; it was still in the planning stages. But the fire had been lit, and about ten minutes after the story came out I called Frank Reese, the godfather of heritage poultry, and told him he had no choice but to get on board—we needed birds for the next Thanksgiving. Frank obliged and took a huge risk by raising eight hundred heritage turkeys for us on his small farm in Kansas.

When the Italian and the US Slow Food boards of directors got wind of the project, they went into panic mode, worried that because we were selling a food item as a profit center, we might jeopardize the nonprofit status of Slow Food USA, or that someone might get sick eating the bird— the very animal we had been celebrating! They also believed that the Ark should not endorse an individual producer. They tried to kill the project.

But it was too late. The shoot-first-think-later approach I had learned from Carlo had already made sure that the sales flyer had gone out to all Slow Food members in the United States. So the directors asked that I start my own company to take full responsibility for the project, which I did, calling it Heritage Foods USA. At first it was the marketing arm of Slow Food USA, but eventually it would grow to be its own self-sustaining business, selling and promoting heritage meat and supporting independent farms.

The project almost crashed a few times—loading hundreds of turkeys onto a FedEx truck in the back of a slaughterhouse was beyond the scope of anything I had been prepared for—but ultimately everyone got their birds and Frank got paid. The second year we sold about fifteen hundred turkeys; the initiative became the most successful

Slow Food operation in the States, and all the profits went to fund Slow Food. Meanwhile, about fifty other farms around the country started to raise heritage turkeys for their local Slow Food *convivia*, great news for our mission to promote biodiversity. At some point the suits on the board of directors seemed to forget that they'd been against the idea from the start.

Many of the farmers who now raised the turkeys with Frank to help meet the sudden demand were calling me, asking if I could help them secure a more regular source of income, since naturally mating turkeys are seasonal, and only available around Thanksgiving. These farmers also raised heritage breeds of pig, cattle, and sheep, as well as ducks and geese. By 2004 Slow Food had grown to more than 11,000 members and 130 chapters, and I was proud that the movement had the infrastructure to survive without me running it. I decided it was time to work directly with independent farmers. In my final letter as the president of Slow Food USA, published in the *Snail,* I invited the membership at large to sign up for my new full-time venture.

The first year we sold everything from half lambs to wild rice to charcuterie, all via FedEx, to home chefs. Then, in the spring of 2005, I took a life-changing trip to visit our family of farms with a small group of believers, including chefs Mark Ladner and Zach Allen from the Mario Batali–Joe Bastianich restaurant group. As expected, they fell in love with the farmers, and with the taste and quality of the meat. Ladner, especially, took a huge leap of faith and said that if we could supply his restaurant Lupa in New York City with pork for six months without fucking up, then the other restaurants in their group—including Babbo and Del Posto and places they were planning to open in Las Vegas and LA—would follow and support us, too.

We ordered our first batch of pigs—Red Wattles, because they were Mark's favorite—and told our farmers to start ramping up production. It was a commitment that would take them years to fulfill because of the slow growth rate of heritage breeds, but we were confident we would succeed and not leave them hanging. Our new partners at Paradise Locker Meats in Trimble, Missouri—whom we met through one of the farmers and have grown to love like family—skillfully cut and processed the meat. Then we found a trucking company, Cannonball Express, to deliver our first few pigs in parts to New York City.

Lupa was mostly buying pork shoulder and jowl, so I started calling my chef friends and cold-calling around to see if anyone would be interested in trying the parts of the pig that Lupa didn't need, including some terrific cuts like bellies, spareribs, hams, and my favorite, the porterhouse chops. The response was amazing, and the next week I found myself hauling ass through the streets of New York in a rented U-Haul van to deliver the meat before it went bad in the summer heat. About a year later we met Pat LaFrieda, the great New York meat distributor, and his right-hand man, Mark Pastore, and we made a great deal with them to deliver our food for us locally. Months later we found a similar delivery service in Northern California, Preferred Meats, owned by Bala Kironde, and Heritage Foods USA really started to hum.

By 2008 we were going through 150 pigs a week, in addition to small numbers of other livestock, not to mention 8,000 turkeys at Thanksgiving. Restaurant groups, including Danny Meyer's Union Square Hospitality Group, signed on for weekly deliveries, as did independent restaurants like Oliveto, A16, and Americano Restaurant at Hotel Vitale in the Bay Area. Then the cure-masters followed and helped us move all the parts of all our pigs. Two of America's great charcutiers—Sam Edwards in Virginia, and Fatted Calf's Taylor Boetticher in California—became our champion customers, transforming our business.

We now deliver to roughly 150 restaurant partners every week, and they are the lifeline for an entire network of independent farms and processors—by supporting heritage breeds and a return to traditional flavors, they are keeping about fifty family-owned businesses up and running. And as our wholesale division expanded to meet a growing demand, we also began to expand our mail-order division, which now sells hundreds of products directly to people's homes, including bison, lamb, goat, and maple syrup.

Today we do much the same thing on the same schedule as we did when we began—pigs are killed on Mondays and Tuesdays while we make sales calls, and then they are cut to order on Wednesdays and Thursdays while we dedicate time to our mail-order division. We do our accounting on Friday, and we work with all the same people we did when we started. Goats, turkeys, ducks, and geese join the fray in October, November, and December. Heritage Foods USA keeps growing, but it never really changes that much—over the years we have learned that the best way to support America's independent farms is to buy from them, and that anything else is bullshit.

———

Since Slow Food began, we have seen fads melt and trends rise and fall. We've seen the food world morph into fashion, where sizzle rules the day no matter where the steak came from.

But the spate of fancy events and color photographs and chef competition shows on television has done little to help American independent farmers sleep at night—or to improve the chances that our planet might survive the current onslaught of corporate farming and the looming realities of climate change. We are drowning in recipes and food porn—when it comes to the real issues that concern our farmers and the health of America's food supply, the food media is failing. It isn't much more than a beauty pageant.

The revolution needed a voice, something to punch through this insipid wall of tawdry, feel-good fluff—so in 2009, largely inspired by Carlo Petrini's 1975 pirate station in Italy, Radio Bra Onde Rosse, we began the Heritage Radio Network, an Internet-based radio station out behind

Roberta's restaurant in Bushwick, Brooklyn. Carlo rescued an old military surplus transmitter to start his station; we built ours out of a couple of recycled shipping containers and put a garden on the roof.

Chris Parachini, Brandon Hoy, and Carlo Mirarchi had opened Roberta's a few months earlier, and were at the vanguard of a new generation of restaurant at once cool and sustainable. Roberta's was unlike any other in America—the restaurant itself was built by the owners themselves out of an old auto body shop with rescued and recycled materials, in an industrial district that nearly burned to the ground during the great blackout of 1977. Now it is very much at the hub of a fantastic new food movement, and the food that comes out of the pizza station and kitchen is delicious. This is also where I met my coauthor, Mike Edison, whose book *I Have Fun Everywhere I Go*—itself a romp through slow culture—had resonated with me. I invited Mike to talk about his work on my radio program, *The Main Course,* and he became a frequent guest and a good friend, eventually beginning his own show.

Heritage Radio now reaches millions of listeners a month. We produce our own content that directly competes with the food coverage on NPR, CNN, and every other major news portal. At the core of the station are thirty fantastic weekly shows—hosted by a diverse group of chefs, authors, visionaries, lunatics, journalists, historians, and hedonists—about food technology, beer, cheese, food history, politics, and cocktails, to name just a few of the myriad, plus a few outlier shows covering alternative music, arts, and pop culture. The station started as something of a clubhouse for subversive foodies but has grown into a legitimate media outlet—we are a source for hard news and opinion, a beacon for like-minded progressives who do not view food as simply fodder for the style section.

————

The first meat question brought up at every sustainable food conference is, without fail, "Should we eat meat, or not?" And my answer is: "Wow, that is one stupid question!" As a nation we sank our teeth into more than ten billion livestock last year. Animals are a huge part of our culture, part of the cycles of agriculture.

The next question we always hear is "How negative are the environmental consequences of meat production? Shouldn't we stop raising cattle for food?" Answer: "Another stupid question!" Since consuming meat is a reality, isn't it better to support a sustainable alternative rather than bleat about an unrealistic vegetarian dream world?

And the final question is always "Can the type of farming you're talking about feed the world?" Well, that's a stupid question, too. The short answer is yes, and it has. That was how the world worked for thousands of years. But given the current situation, more or less owned by industrial farming, which is not feeding the whole world, either, we should focus on small victories and get back to the garden, as they say.

THE CARNIVORE'S MANIFESTO carves a path for eating meat and living well on the planet Earth—it is a declaration of principles and a guide for day-to-day living. Every one of the essays in this book is a call to arms. And everything in this book is doable. Some chapters call for aggressive changes in the Industrial Food Complex; others put forth changes that can be made in your kitchens and pantries and local markets. A few essays were even given voice by our animal friends themselves.

Our lives are better when we make the right choices through a heightened awareness of the world around us—of farmers and truck drivers and burger flippers and bartenders and of the food on the supermarket shelves; of our relationship to technology and nature, and especially, ultimately, to what's at the end of our forks—and so we offer an uncompromised manifesto based on real experience. Our goal is to break the trend of fewer companies producing the majority of what America eats; to have more people and more farms producing more of our food; and to move away from shamelessly irresponsible commodity products to a healthy, high-quality alternative, no matter where you live, no matter what you do.

Eating better meat will be more expensive. But perhaps as quality replaces cheap commodity, some people will end up eating less meat—which is not such a bad thing. We are fighting for healthy diets and better lives, not for rampant, Paleolithic pig roasts every night of the week. And while we think meat is an important component of a healthy human diet, we aren't just carnivore, we're omnivore, and if that includes eating a Mallomar once in a while, at least we know exactly what we are putting in our mouths.

THE CARNIVORE'S MANIFESTO represents a slow turning of the screw, a process that is greased with great joy. It was born of action, for people who are ready to become leaders, each in their own way, in charge of their own sustainable, fair, and rewarding food destiny, whether that means sleeping with your butcher, or simply laying off the Happy Meals.

The message is simple. Enjoy your life. Eat great meat. Use this book to create your own revolution.

Patrick Martins

Brooklyn, New York, May 2013

CHAPTER 1

A Is for Apprentice

Hard work ain't easy, but it's fair.
—*Larry Holmes*

Sometimes there is nothing like getting hit in the face.

When it comes to boxing, this is what it takes to be a champ: thousands of hours of roadwork and brutal training, thousands of hours of learning to focus and throwing a million punches, working the speed bag, the heavy bag, sparring, and learning to duck and weave. But no matter what, you are going to get hit, and hit hard, and learn the hard realities of your chosen profession; even seasoned veterans and experts have something to learn.

Thomas Odermatt in San Francisco has been perfecting the same porchetta sandwich on a food truck, the Roli Roti, for twelve years, and I'd put my money on it as the best sandwich in America because he knows there is no such thing as a perfect sandwich—the apex of crunchiness and the ephemeral balance of spices, meat, skin, and attendant grease—the best he can do is make a sandwich that only suggests what perfection might be like if God allowed it to exist. Striving for it is his noble purpose.

Cruz Goler has been the head chef at Lupa for more than six years and claims he cannot make the restaurant's signature *cacio e pepe* pasta perfectly every time—it's too simple, there are only four ingredients, the margin of error is too small. Sean Heller, the former chef at Momofuku Noodle Bar, said the same thing about making the simple ramen noodle—it's a humbling experience every time he makes it.

Up until 1835, a butcher in New York City had to work at least five years chopping meat before he could legitimately call himself a butcher, and for his effort and skill he'd earn a seal with the emblem of his craft, which he could put on his storefront to signify that he was the real deal.

What does it take to become a master sushi chef? How many hours do you have to spend with that knife in your hands? Japanese culture is much more patient than American culture—we are always in a rush and chasing trends, and sometimes we forget about quality.

What is the difference between being a bar band and the E Street Band? Or between busking and playing with the New York Philharmonic? And what's the difference between playing in the string section in the extended complement of the orchestra and sitting in the first-violin chair?

Do you really think it's just raw talent? The Beatles slugged it out in Hamburg playing three sets a night to the toughest crowds imaginable before they got to record "She Loves You," and even then they were turned down by more than a dozen record companies. As the saying goes, they worked years to become overnight sensations. Pretty singing is nice, but nothing can replace playing two thousand sets of music.

How is it that Michael Jordan, one of the greatest athletes of all time, could only muster a batting average a few cents above .200 when he decided he wanted to play baseball? And that was in the minor leagues! It's because he didn't spend twenty years swinging the lumber every day. Hitting a baseball is very difficult—Derek Jeter, arguably the most talented Yankee of his generation, has been swinging a bat every day since he was three and he *still* had to spend a few seasons down on the farm before he got called up to The Show.

Swinging a bat and playing Paganini, like cooking, are activities that dispose quickly of the notion that consistency is the hobgoblin of little minds—just think of what it takes to make the perfectly poached egg, every time, without fail. You can't learn that in a class one morning and then expect to deliver the goods on the highest level every day without ever making a mess of it.

The tradition of apprenticeship in the United States has largely been replaced by colleges and the university system. One problem with this is that it is mostly a pay-to-play scenario. School can be wildly expensive, but the revolution needs to be open to everyone, especially the industrious—and by the way, that is my favorite word. *Industrious*. It describes to me a quality that should always trump who you know or where you went to school.

Somewhere along America's journey we have lost the importance of apprenticeship and the idea of what it means to spend ten thousand hours with a knife in your hands, or ten thousand hours baking bread, or five years burning your hands and sweating it out on the line under a master chef and sucking it up until you can graduate to journeyman, and then—years later—to master, and then open your own place.

This restaurant business is high-risk and rife with failure, but look at the people who have been in the racket for a long time, the masters, and check out their failure-to-success ratio—I'm talking about Danny Meyer, Tom Colicchio, Joe Bastianich, and Mario Batali, among others. They paid their dues coming up, and now they almost always go twelve rounds and leave with the belt. That's not luck, that's not celebrity, that's old-school experience.

I was speaking at Yale recently and an enthusiastic young man asked me how to get into the beer world, but when pressed he had to confess that he had never actually tried to brew anything! He was so out there he asked me what kind of beer he should start with. I told him "How about a lager? And quit holding your nose up at Budweiser." Sure, it is industrially brewed, but it is the classic American lager, thirst-quenching, satisfying, honest, fulfills its own promise, and is remarkably consistent. Work on *that* for five years, and then maybe you can start fooling around with a hemp-infused porter.

Our culture rewards youth far too quickly. We tend to shut out old actors—sadly, especially women. In music, if you haven't made it by the time you're twenty-four you might as well forget it. Bob Dylan already sounded like an old man when he was a teenager, but if he had recorded his first record when he was fifty, do you think anyone would have noticed? Old dancers get moved out for young ballerinas who might leap a bit higher, but can they move an entire audience with a subtle gesture of their hands, nuances of the art that can only be learned across a lifetime? It angers me to think how quickly we dismiss our master craftspeople to make room for the Next Big Thing. Remember that in the martial arts it is considered a privilege for a neophyte to be beaten by someone with color on their belt.

And this is why, for all the talk about "artisanal," we are losing the sense of *art*. Look at Picasso, or Kandinsky— when they had their epiphanies they had thrown around enough paint to be able to execute their vision. They weren't masters, but they were masters of figure studies and the quick sketch. Matisse and de Kooning spent so much time with pencils in their hands that when it came time to do their own thing they didn't trip over technique. Before Jackson Pollock started slinging paint, he studied with Thomas Hart Benton and spent four years working for the WPA's Federal Art Project. All of them paid their dues with the equity of sweat. And all of these artists were smart enough to know that they would never know it all; their quest for knowledge was positively *rabbinical,* even after they had reached summits others only dream of.

We would do well to foster a system where sweat is rewarded as much as cleverness, a return to valuing the working class, and to rewarding the elevation of art through practical experience. We need to get back to celebrating mundane, hard work. Consistency in execution, and the exalted handing down of knowledge. Repetition toward perfection. The flawlessly efficient guitar solo. The perfect sandwich. The knockout blow.

CHAPTER 2

The $140 Turkey

What is a cynic? A man who knows the price of
everything and the value of nothing.

—*Oscar Wilde*

Is this book elitist? Are we wrong and living some entitled,
aristocratic fantasy when we demand that *everyone* eat better, cleaner, and more responsible meat?

If you think so, then you are waging a class war. You
are saying that quality food is not an issue for poor people.

No one deserves to eat unhealthy meat. And all of our
children deserve to eat healthy farm-raised food, in the
same way they deserve love and affection and a safe
environment.

Right now we are looking at the first generation in centuries whose life-span is predicted to be shorter than that of
their parents, threatened by obesity and a host of hor-
rifying health issues. Not advocating for fresh, healthy,

sustainable meat for everyone, and especially for children —
even if it costs more — is like putting a discount liquor store
in every urban neighborhood. It's like looking the other
way when drug dealers infiltrate housing projects. It rein-
forces the very worst of a broken socioeconomic hierarchy
and only serves to advance the most pronounced social
problems.

Do you think I am a spoiled, rich foodie for selling $140
turkeys — or that I am ripping people off because you can
get a $20 turkey at the supermarket? If that turkey suffered,
if its biosystem was compromised by genetic tomfoolery,
and antibiotics, and if the farm behind the bird pollutes the
planet with chemicals and animal waste and shrugs when
paying the fine, and you are still basting it come Thanksgiving Day, you are an accessory to a crime.

Still, do you think promoting good meat is elitist? And
if you do, I ask, how do you presume that commodity meat
is as safe and nutritious as natural meat? How do you put
them on the same level? How can you be so blind to the
differences?

There is a mentality that spending $500 to see a Rolling
Stones concert is a righteous thing, while buying a $140 tur-
key is throwing money away. But unlike inflated concert
ticket prices, $140 represents the true cost of raising that
bird naturally and getting it delivered, and you can bet that
the farmer who raised it isn't getting rich on it.

Bringing quality food to all Americans must be our
shared goal. We understand that it might not always be

accessible and easily affordable, but the argument that a diet of fresh food is somehow elitist must die right now.

I love Michel Nischan and Gus Schumacher's Wholesome Wave initiative, which fosters strong linkages between local agriculture and underserved communities. Their Double Value Coupon Program doubles the buying power of federal nutrition benefits (food stamps) at farmers' markets, encouraging people to eat fresh fruit and vegetables while supporting local farmers. Their program started with just a few participants, but after less than five years they are working with three thousand farms in twenty-eight states, and everyone in the program is eating more fresh food, and buying it at farmers' markets and not corporate supermarkets.

So what's the true cost of that cheap bird that hurts the planet and is unhealthy for everyone who comes into contact with it, from the worker on the farm to the kid who eats it for lunch?

It's time to stop arguing for the consumption of unhealthy and suffering animals. The $140 turkey is a robust, healthy animal that lived a great life, and by the time that gorgeous meat gets to your plate it costs about $8 for a portion with a potato and some organic greens—not much more than dinner at McDonald's.

CHAPTER 3

To Hell with Local, Eat the Best

Taste, like identity, has meaning only when there is difference.

—*Carlo Petrini*

Sadly, calling yourself a *locavore* has become a virulent strain of fascistic fashion, an *haute couture* chimera for foodie snarks and uptight hippies.

Remember this: *Local* is a measurement of distance, not of taste. The idea of eating locally sourced food is admirable, but too quickly it has become all about geography, not gastronomy.

Slow Food was never originally about eating locally; it is about eating the best and preserving and celebrating the unique traits that come to food from a specific region and its producers. Traditionally, the best anchovies come from Sicily, the best *bottarga* from Sardinia, the best lentils from

Puy, France. There are great and varied eggplants from all over the world, and no, they are not interchangeable.

New York is good for apples, but peaches, not so much. Maybe one hundred years ago you had no choice other than inferior local produce, but the world is a much smaller place now. If it is peaches you want, look to central Georgia, the Ojai Valley, or western Michigan, or any place whose climate is suited to growing peaches. To force that on New York is not geographically or environmentally efficient, or even gastronomically preferable. It's folly.

My friends in Oregon are proud of their backyard truffles, but seriously? I know pigs that refuse to hunt for them. The point is that anytime you reward a local *terroir* over actual taste, you are doing a disservice to your taste buds, and ultimately to the local farmer by propping up a fifth-rate product. No points are given for geography, otherwise I would just graze in my backyard.

American food is wonderful, but if this country is ever going to rise to the gastronomic heights of France, Italy, and Spain, and take strides toward global respect for our national cuisine, we must begin to see our country as a unified gastronomic mosaic and acknowledge brilliance where it exists. Who would argue that Georgia produces a one-of-a-kind Vidalia onion that is practically like candy, or that the Southwest is ground zero for smoky chilis? Why do my friends in San Francisco, Portland, Orlando, Madrid, London, and pretty much everywhere else ask me to stuff a dozen New York bagels into my carry-on when I come to visit? Because local water and baking at sea level (not to mention our shared Jewish experience) make the New York bagel a bauble that cannot be improved on.

I love cheddar cheese from New York state and Vermont, but there is no better grating cheese than Parmigiano-Reggiano off the boat from Italy. I drink wine from all over the world, but never from Brooklyn. However, we make great beer here. And yet different beer occasions require different beers—why shouldn't I enjoy a rainy-afternoon pint of Guinness? Maybe when they open a brewery run by Trappist monks in Bushwick I'll drink their ale when I want something sweet. Until then, it's Chimay for me. And while you are ooohing and aaahing about the locally sourced honey, be aware that you could be denying yourself pleasure in the misguided pursuit of politically correct gastronomy. Some bees and some flowers make for better honey than others—and personally, I try to avoid anything that pollinates within spitting distance of the Brooklyn-Queens Expressway.

We've been through a powerful revolution in America. Over the last thirty years, food has gotten better everywhere. But the local food movement and the do-it-yourselfers have to open their minds to the best-tasting alternatives, even if they are from another planet. Local is awesome, but until it's the best in the land, trust your mouth, not the map.

CHAPTER 4

Learn to Build a Fire

Yet, as only New Yorkers know, if you can get
through the twilight, you'll live through the night.
— *Dorothy Parker*

For all the technological prowess we possess, most of us
would be clueless without the help of the most basic of
tools — for instance, a Swiss Army knife, a refrigerator, or a
pack of matches.

For all our fantastic knowledge of computers and communication, if we were whisked back in a time a century or
two, what could we bring, in the style of Prometheus, to
our new contemporaries? We could tell them about pho-
tography and recorded sound and the miracle of radio and
television, but not one in a million of us could actually build
anything to demonstrate such magic, let alone "invent" any
of those things and get rich based on the know-how of our
future selves.

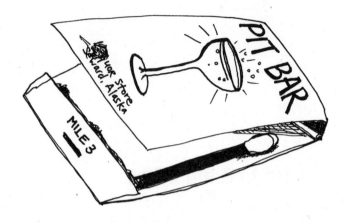

More importantly, could you build shelter? Hunt for food, or fish? Could you build a fire to cook, keep you warm, and protect yourself from varmints?

Control of fire—one of two primary ingredients in any meat dish—is one of those things that represent behavioral modernity. Cavemen were aces at it. And yet here we are, only marginally impressed that we have successfully sent a robot to Mars, but we'd be shit out of luck if we ended up like Tom Hanks in *Cast Away,* or one of the kids in *Lord of the Flies.*

You can bet that in the formative years of America, everyone learned at least one skill that helped them survive: how to kill and dress a deer. Build a house. Navigate by the stars. Identify edible and poisonous plants. Milk a cow and make butter. Build a fire.

Part of THE CARNIVORE'S MANIFESTO is a call to celebrate the bounty of the earth and the power of nature before it was hijacked by the Industrial Revolution. Everyone, every person on the planet, uses fire in some way, every day, whether the fire is for making tea or internally combusting inside the crosstown bus.

Fire is the prime mover in that thing called cooking, and it is just one more miracle we take for granted. And when the lights go off—they have before and they will again—the firestarter will be as a king.

CHAPTER 5

Survival of the Fattest

There are no shortcuts in evolution.
—*Louis D. Brandeis*

Sad But True Department: The turkey traditionally "pardoned" by the president in a White House pre-Thanksgiving ritual is known for dropping dead without any help, just weeks after its big photo op.

Generally, the turkeys presented are the usual suspect, the Broad Breasted White, the omnipresent product of corporate overbreeding. Much like all birds and livestock raised on factory farms, the Broad Breasted White is a cut-and-paste collage of genetic engineering.

Corporate turkeys cannot survive in nature. Their cardiovascular systems can hardly support their outsized bodies. Their muscles and bones are weak. Their immune system has been so compromised by genetic monkey-wrenching that they need to be fed antibiotics just to make it to the pardon.

Factory animal farms started to breed for genetic *deformities* in the 1970s. In an odd reversal of the master-race ideals of Nazis, who dreamed of weeding out the weak, corporate Dr. Frankensteins scoured flocks and herds of animals, millions of them, over years, looking for the misfits. Deformities that ranked highest on the Corporate Farming Most Wanted list included abnormally fast growth rate and feed conversion, large breasts, short legs, and stupidity—these were the traits that would help the bottom line.

When they came across one of nature's mistakes—say, a chicken so top-heavy with meat that it could barely walk—they pulled it from the flock, not to kill it in an effort to protect the group from bad genes, but to ensure that its abnormal genetics became part of the next year's harvest.

The misfits were cataloged and combined—corporate farms now consist of entire populations whose skeletal, cardiovascular, and immune systems can't keep up with their genetic engineering. Long before they got to the crowded feeding ops, these animals were doomed to a life of pain with a potpourri of scurrilous genetics.

But boy, do they grow fast! A twenty-pound turkey has gone from taking twenty-four weeks to only twelve weeks to fully grow, but many are on the verge of collapse when they arrive on the kill floor. Factory farming methods have cut two months off the natural growing time of a pig, and 25 percent off the time it takes cattle to get to kill weight—but these animals get sick easily. If you grew as fast as a corporate chicken, you would weigh 349 pounds at age two. Congratulations, Pilgrim's, Tyson, Perdue, Wayne Farms, House of Raeford, Keystone Foods, and Koch Foods, among others—you have created a race of freaks! Heart failure and sudden death are now common—a 5 percent death rate in chickens is now considered a success.

Good, clean, and fair farms also breed for certain traits, but the philosophy behind what they are doing is the old philosophy of balance. Their ideal animal is one that is healthy, strong, and capable of reproducing and foraging, and lives a long time. Selective breeding, as opposed to genetic engineering, ensures the foundation for a humanely raised, healthy animal, one that might actually benefit from a presidential pardon.

CHAPTER 6

Commodity vs. Quality

People seldom do what they believe in. They do
what is convenient, then repent.

—*Bob Dylan*

Imagine a world where everything is the same, where even
the giant box of sixty-four Crayola crayons—the magic box
that fractured the spectrum into such treasures as periwin-
kle, fuchsia, and burnt sienna—has been reduced to one dull
monotone, and one made of inferior but cheap-to-produce
wax, all in the name of efficiency and profit margins. What a
sad place that would be.

This is the world where commodity has finally taken
over. But how far away from that humdrum dystopia are we?

We are a nation fixed on commodities and hooked on
convenience. Too often we shop solely motivated by price
points that can only be maintained by corporate economies
of the grandest scale.

One of the problems with commodity goods—products resulting from the lowest common denominator and the strategy of fast-faster-fastest, the attitude that drives the global economy—is that the price never reflects the true cost of the goods being traded, such as the impact on the environment and fair labor practices.

The real problem is that cheap shit breaks, and the nuisance it causes far outweighs any up-front savings, and largely, you can't fix something that was mass-produced. It just needs to be replaced.

Quality may seem more expensive when you're at the checkout counter, but quality isn't about cost, it's about value. Quality is patient. Quality takes the long view. Quality takes time, and is evident by its lasting character.

There is always the acceptable low end of any product—not every car can be a Bentley, not every guitar a genuine Les Paul—but the sign of a commodity, on the other hand, is that it is made and marketed to be the cheapest version of its kind, mass-produced with a disdain for differentiation and a lust for low cost and high profit. And so we get cars that break down, and guitars that look pretty from a distance but can't stay in tune.

Which is why commodity food, and especially meat, sucks. It is against everything this book advocates and celebrates. Commodity in the food world is the exact opposite of slow food.

A commodity by its very definition should approach

zero qualitative differentiation across the market. A commodity is fungible, as the economists like to say, meaning that the market doesn't care who the producer is, and the less signature, meaning the less you can tell anything apart, the better. Personal style, charming inconsistencies, local flavor, anything original, exceptional, or even marginally unique needs to be removed. "From the taste of wheat it is not possible to tell who produced it, a Russian serf, a French peasant, or an English capitalist," Karl Marx once mused.

Once upon a time, the concept of commodity in food was intended to make certain that farmers were paid a fair price even in bad years. In eighteenth-century Japan the shogunate set a price for rice that would assure farmers and everyone involved in the supply chain, from delivery men to merchants, a living wage, and guarantee that everyone — including the samurai, who were paid in rice — could afford to eat.

But these days, the "going rate" — the market price of a commodity — is manipulated by the robber barons of Wall Street, likely in collusion with Big Ag, which games the system to maximize profits, crushing small family farms in the process. This numbers game favors output and gross intake over the more intangible yet enduring qualities of satisfaction, reputation, and legacy, not to mention what is actually good for you.

Efficiency is admirable. However, when efficiency is championed over quality or safety in food, when profit margin pushes for chickens that grow like weeds but are so sick they need to be juiced with an ocean of chemicals just so they don't die before we kill them, we all suffer.

The ins and outs of trading food commodities are sophisticated and difficult for anyone without a degree in economics to parse. But know that the kind of commodity trading that Goldman Sachs and its peers practice has helped push food prices to historic highs—money that never reaches the independent farmer—and has been a major factor in worldwide food shortages. Hunger is a justice issue, not a poverty issue, as my friend Tony Butler, the executive director of Bread and Life, likes to say.

We want to see all consumers take other factors into consideration besides price per pound when they buy food, and understand that anyone who buys commodity goods is basically complicit in their crimes. If an industrial farmer is dumping poison in a river and paying a relative pittance of a fine as part of "the cost of doing business," and you're still frying his chickens, you are part of the problem.

It's time we stopped using money as a shield for the barons of industrial farming—the claim that healthy meat is too expensive, or that poor people can't afford it, must be squashed. Our goal should be to feed everyone the best food possible, even if we eat less. We demand a new commodity rate for sustainable meat, for food that is healthy and produced not in factories but on farms. All people have the right to eat this way.

CHAPTER 7

Slow Food Is Fast Food

Re-examine all you have been told...dismiss that
which insults your soul.

—*Walt Whitman*

We're sick of hearing about people braising a pork shoulder for twenty hours. With so much time spent cooking, who the hell has time to eat? No wonder our local farms are going out of business!

And recipes? Enough already. Please! Does the world really need another reimagining of *boeuf bourguignon?* What we need is better beef. Do you really think you can improve on a California strawberry picked at the peak of its sweetness? Do carrots need to be dosed with enough herbs to make them trip? Not if they're good carrots.

And that's the worst part of the sort of overcomplicated cooking that has become fashionable, these romanticized home science projects—it has taken over the most important part of our gastronomic experience. Alice Waters says that 90 percent of cuisine is agriculture, and our job is not to obliterate the essence of our food by cooking it so much that the component parts become unrecognizable.

Slow food is not about extended cooking techniques or complex recipes; it's about quality ingredients. It's about sourcing responsibly, recognizing the farmer's work, and understanding exactly what we are eating and where it comes from. Whether it's a rib eye or a radish, the important thing is the provenance, not the preparation.

Sure, sometimes you want to make dinner a culinary flight of fancy, the Mardi Gras parade of flavors, but if we were to make a big deal out of preparation every time we wanted to get with the knife and fork, we'd never get to eat! Slow food is about the quotidian. It's not a fantasy; it's what's for dinner.

Why do so-called foodies feel the need to applaud and get out their camera phones every time a plate is put in front of them? Isn't it enough to have a fresh piece of fish cooked well—even if it took no prep and the only ingredient other than the fish is fire? Well, okay, maybe some sea salt and fresh pepper, some good olive oil, a lemon if there is one skulking around, but you get the point. The fish did its job; it doesn't want you to hide it in some fancy sauce.

To make slow food work as a movement and as a practical lifestyle choice, we have to treat it like *fast* food. Basically, don't think about it, eat it! Have a beautiful piece of meat? Apply heat, *et voilà*. Sure, a little nuance with a skillet never hurt, but there is no reason to complicate things when you want to eat. Cooking a good piece of meat and steaming some vegetables (let alone eating them raw) takes less time than ordering Chinese takeout, which in New York, I have been told, is cooked by a guy on a bicycle on his way over to your apartment.

If you came to my house for dinner, would you be disappointed if I served a perfectly grilled heritage pork chop that came from a very happy pig that lived a wonderful life? To do it right, it takes about eight minutes from heat to plate. The slow part happened before I even got that chop home.

An apple is slow food. A jar of organic peanut butter is slow food. Chili made with turkey ground from a heritage bird, fresh tomatoes, and organic beans is slow food. Take this attitude and you'll eat better food—convenient and quick doesn't have to mean junk. I guarantee you, it will be better than any meal you can get in a "family" restaurant, and at a fraction of the cost.

In America food shopping has become a function of convenience, but increasingly even large chain stores are offering organic options. Walmart has gotten into the game, and of course if you live in New York or Los Angeles or Chicago or San Francisco or anywhere where there are slightly affluent hippies or hipsters, there are going to be lots of places that specialize in responsibly sourced food. If you want it, it's all there.

We need to eighty-six forever the idea that healthy is

haughty. Slow food is simple. Slow food is humble. Slow food is fast. It's everyday. Remember: A healthy burger from cattle raised on the tallgrass prairies of Oklahoma takes no more time to flip than the sad meat patty they serve at McDonald's.

CHAPTER 8

Merchants Matter

We make a living by what we get, but we make a
life by what we give.

— *Winston Churchill*

Once upon a time there was a merchant class. Sometimes
it was exalted — the Medici family rose from textile merchants to bankers to a cabal that chose the Pope — and
sometimes disdained, as in China, where merchants are
perceived as profiting off mere trade, not actually creating
anything and exploiting the labor and craftsmanship of
others.

The basic definition of a merchant is one who trades in
goods that are produced by others. Some merchants are
noble in their pursuits, great distributors of culture. Unfortunately, some are simply useless middlemen — the American cliché of a fast-talking broker who has his hand out and
makes money by cutting corners, price-gouging, lying

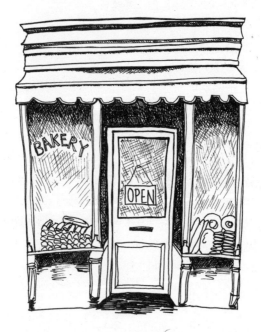

about the source, and generally baiting, switching, taking the money, and then taking off.

My wife is one of the good ones. She's a cheesemonger, and you can find her in her shop or warehouse every day, representing the goods she has personally selected to wear her seal of approval. Caputo's deli on Court Street in Brooklyn sells wonderful Italian delicacies that the owners have a real connection to—the owners are the ones making the sandwiches, and they are as intimate with every one of the hundreds of ingredients in their cases as they are with their clientele.

And this is who we are talking about: the merchant who sits in his (or her) own shop and knows his customers.

This is about the purveyor who cares, who buys and resells thoughtfully. This is about the guy who travels the world looking for the very best, the merchant whose name unequivocally means quality. I am one of those guys—this is what connects you and me. You want to eat humanely sourced, naturally raised, chemical-free meat of an exceedingly high standard, and I am the guy who knows the farmers and who can bring their products to you responsibly and for a fair price. I work hard to earn your trust.

Steve Jenkins of Fairway Market is a big reason I chose to become a merchant. Ariane Daguin is another great New York–based merchant. She is my competitor and I respect her. Ariane, who along with George Faison founded D'Artagnan, is among the finest purveyors of French-style meat products. From foie gras to Toulouse geese to country pâté to truffles—everything they touch is first class, and as with Heritage, you can trust the people behind their brand.

People like this are at the forefront of what is still a noble merchant class, and I am proud to be part of it. I take a lot of pride in all of my suppliers. I know them all personally. We work closely together—it is very difficult for a midsized independent farmer to get his or her product to market without my infrastructure. Likewise, my business depends on them, just as it depends on treating the diner who eventually puts the meat in his or her mouth with respect. Nothing less will do.

On the other hand, corporate food purveyors and industrial farmers, not to put too fine a point on it, do not give a flying fuck. They don't need you. They compete on price and convenience and rely on a largely passive and undiscerning public. When you move billions in processed meat every year, one customer doesn't even rate as a voice in the wilderness. Big food corporations, after all, are not really in the food business, they are in the money business. That's why you should never buy your food from publicly traded companies.

That's a pretty big rule to try to follow, and given the realpolitik of this book, we aren't going to wield that hammer too despotically, because eventually we are going to want some Mallomars (Mondelēz International), or some Gatorade (PepsiCo). But don't ever forget that a corporation's goal is to make profits, as much and as quickly as possible, period—not an ideal model for selling quality food.

In historic times it was the Medicis and the Rothschilds who rode the high seas to foreign lands to bring back merchandise for eager consumers. They put their family crest on every product they sold. Once upon a time, kings paid merchants to go out on ships and risk their lives, to come back years later with silks and jewels and cacao and tobacco.

Marco Polo is one of my heroes. I love the romance of the merchant traveler. My version of the Silk Road is paved with pork chops. I went to Kansas City in 2004—to expand Heritage Foods USA beyond just turkeys—and made handshake agreements with farmers and slaughterhouses, and the next week there was a pallet of meat that I took to kitchens in New York. I mortgaged everything—there was no safety net. Back in New York, we were fortunate—like Marco Polo returning to Venice—to have fantastic consumers who really knew the difference between commodity and quality.

If I tried to start cutting costs to boost my margin, or squeezing farmers harder, everyone would know it in a hot second. My business would be over. No matter how big a customer you are, one bad piece of meat and I've lost you.

Big Ag spends more money lobbying the government to keep regulators off its backs than all my farmers put together make in profit from selling healthy food. Big Ag's responsibility is not to anyone but its stockholders, who obviously, empirically, don't worry themselves about ramifications—locally, globally, or spiritually. In the last decade, industrial chicken farmers paid more money in fines for dumping toxic waste into a river than Heritage Food might earn in my lifetime. But you know, according to them, poisoning the planet—well, being caught doing it, anyway—is part of the price of doing business.

Can you imagine what would happen if I ever did anything that was even remotely environmentally unsound? Game over. We don't hide anything—we list every one of our farms and vendors, and every restaurant that serves or sells our product, on our website. Obviously, we take pride in every one of them.

Quality merchants are real people. Corporations are faceless and inaccessible. They are arrogant. Just try getting Jim Perdue on the phone to discuss antibiotics in his feed or how his livestock are treated, or why there was a class-action suit brought against his company—by the Humane Society of the United States, in a federal court in New Jersey, where the society represented consumers who were being "duped" by Perdue's false claims—the very second he started asserting that his chickens were "humanely raised."

Got a problem with Heritage Foods USA? Or love what we do? Call me. My number is 718-389-0985.

CHAPTER 9

Bessie and Babe, Fluffy and Fido

You think we'd have cattle if people didn't eat 'em every day? They'd just be funny-lookin' animals in zoos.

—*Temple Grandin*

No has done more to fight for the rights of animals than Temple Grandin. She is the voice for those who cannot speak, namely our friends in the animal kingdom. Grandin suffers from autism. One result of her disorder is that she sees the world in pictures, in much the same way animals do. Rather than limit her capabilities, this way of looking at the world has inspired her to write numerous books, including *Thinking in Pictures* and our favorite, *Animals Make Us Human*. Grandin's story is so compelling that Claire Danes played her in a recent Hollywood biopic.

Grandin has used her uncanny ability to think visually and to see things that other humans cannot, to help better the lives of animals, especially livestock during their final trip to the abattoir. She literally got down on hands and knees and crawled through the pens and slaughter chutes just as the animals do, and she learned, among many other things, that the effect of bright lights, deafening noise, and 90-degree turns along the path to their final moment was terrorizing, and that it wasn't just cruel, it was bad for business.

Her insights led her to become a consultant within the Industrial Food Complex for large companies like McDonald's and Cargill, who finally understood that the mandate to make the slaughterhouse a less traumatic experience wasn't just a liberal notion from animal activists, it made financial sense: Stressed animals make bad meat, "dark cutter" beef, and soft, exudative pork, for example. It was nothing short of an incredible accomplishment for a woman with such considerable challenges to break through a male-dominated corporate culture that was averse to any sort of change.

Grandin helped design better animal-handling facilities, including an ingenious series of restraints, chutes, ramps, and stunning systems that were far more humane than the previous status quo—and she continues to push for cameras on kill floors.

"I believe that the best way to create good living conditions for any animal," she wrote in *Animals Make Us Human*, "whether it's a captive animal living in a zoo, a farm animal or a pet, is to base animal welfare programs on the core emotion systems in the brain. My theory is that the environment animals live in should activate their positive emotions as much as possible, and not activate their negative emotions any more than necessary. If we get the animal's emotions right, we will have fewer problem behaviors.... All animals and people have the same core emotion systems in the brain."

For all of God's creatures, from Bessie and Babe to Fluffy and Fido to every one of us, a mind is a terrible thing to waste. And like humans, animals have a basic impulse to search, investigate, and make sense of the environment. Largely, they need to *seek*.

Seeking brings with it the pleasure of thinking that something good is about to come. It brings excitement. It gets the brain waves going. And when you stifle an animal's ability to seek, it will go stir-crazy, and can lash out with rage, or become severely depressed. On the other hand, animals—like humans—that are active are healthier, stronger, more productive, and more intelligent.

For a chicken, seeking can be having room to give itself a dust bath. Or playing with a string, which is like a day at Six Flags for most of them. Turkeys need to pick around for their food, an instinct that is not possible to fulfill because of the barbaric industrial practice of beak clipping. Turkeys should also be allowed to roost and fly, God-given rights they lose on the factory farm. Pigs need to root with their snouts and explore their surroundings—their desire to seek is almost hyperactive. This is why sow stalls are so especially sad. Cows need the freedom of pasture. Also, the stress of weaning a calf at too young an age, common practice in industrial agriculture, kills the desire to seek.

Seeking is also a phenomenon of dogs and cats. Dogs need to investigate new things, chase, play, and exercise. They were bred to be human companions, so leaving a dog at home alone for the workday five days a week is a crime. Would you leave your son or daughter locked in a room all day long? We're not necessarily equating children with pets, but they are often closer than we think.

Cats need to hunt and prowl, and need an outlet for the very curiosity that is eventually going to kill them—they need to use up all nine lives. And although they can be great independent spirits, socialized cats almost always thrive better when they have companions.

Zoos must be held to the same standards. Nomadic hunting animals like polar bears have a tough time adjusting to life in captivity no matter how much they are pampered. Gus, the famous polar bear in the Central Park Zoo in New York City, actually had to see a therapist for a while. Zoos that don't do everything possible to make sure their animals are engaged and happy deserve the wrath of the entire animal kingdom.

We're not advocating for chicken condos or doggy vacation villas, or group encounter sessions for sows, but it is time to stop all the torture even in its less obvious forms,

like inhibiting animals' curiosity. All animals, from livestock raised for food to zoo animals, to our pets, which we
welcome as family members, are part of our humanity, but
they have no voice of their own. We owe it to them to walk
a mile in their paws.

CHAPTER 10

Night of the Hunter

I think anyone who is a carnivore needs to understand that meat does not originally come in these
neat little packages.
—*Julia Child*

Most people will never see how the meat gets to their
mouths. They can't, or won't, imagine how a cow or a pig
gets turned into burger or bacon. But that's not something
you can say about the folks who go out and kill their own.

Too many of us who live in urban jungles are so far
removed from the primacy of our food that we've come to
the cosmopolitan conclusion that putting a bullet or an
arrow into an animal is somehow repulsive, even as we
pull the shrink-wrap off a supermarket steak that was born
of a corporate culture reeking of cruelty and chemicals.

Hunting is noble and pure of purpose. It is our legacy—
we were hunters and gatherers for tens of thousands of

years before the idea of a farm ever took hold. As a source of meat, hunting is the shortest distance between two points, a much better option than the reality of factory-farmed food, which still hovers in the ether of Upton Sinclair's worst nightmare.

Unfortunately, too many of our left-wing liberal elite friends have become zero-tolerance reactionaries when it comes to guns—oh, how they would like to see them all turned into plowshares!

But let it be said, right here and without any ambiguity, that we are not part of that group. THE CARNIVORE'S MANIFESTO is prohunting. And most Americans agree with us.

And that's why the NRA really puts a bee in our bonnet when it insists on falsely connecting America's desire to remove assault rifles from our streets with some nonexistent slope of the slippery variety that ends with the government going house to house to remove guns legally purchased for hunting.

The NRA is ridiculous and dangerous. Its leadership is irresponsible and amoral. It purposely conflates moderate, reasonable gun control with the opinions of a small group of antigun extremists, and, disguised as a group of patriots, plays to the fears of Americans with specious reasoning and outright lies. The NRA does not represent America, it represents greedy weapons manufacturers who put profit for product sold above the safety of our children.

We believe strongly that guns should be registered. We believe in background checks and mandatory waiting periods. We believe that no one needs an assault rifle, or a firearm larger than LeBron James. We are quite certain that civilians do not need armor-piercing ammo, or extended clips, or large-load magazines. And although it is difficult to deny that we'd look pretty hot driving around Brooklyn in a tank, we are going to abstain from such flamboyance for the good of, well, everyone. We abhor anyone who would kill simply for sport. We loathe poachers and the hunters of any protected species.

But responsible hunters are truly at the heart of the sustainable food movement. They eat what they kill. They use every part of the animal. They understand the cycle of life and the ebb and flow of nature in a way nonhunters will never understand.

Love the hunter — for that is who we are.

CHAPTER 11

Têtoir: Feed Your Head

Well done is better than well said.

—*Benjamin Franklin*

A tree may grow in Brooklyn, but Brooklyn will never be known for its *terroir*.

What Brooklyn is known for is its *attitude* and its *culture*, a distinctive accent in everything it does, from pizza to Shooting the Freak at Coney Island, and more recently to starring as a key player in a new food revolution. Brooklyn is a breeding ground for all sorts of art and music, as well as the homestead for some of America's best working writers.

In a word, Brooklyn is a hotbed of *têtoir*.

Têtoir is a word I made up, from the word *tête*, which is French for head. *Têtoir* is similar to *terroir*—what *terroir* is to the earth, *têtoir* is to the mind.

Terroir describes the characteristics that a place imparts to a food made from agricultural products, most famously wine but including everything from fruits and vegetables to coffee and tea to grass-fed meat and honey. Rainfall, drainage, sunlight, day and night temperature differentials, soil type, length of seasons, indigenous life, proximity to large bodies of water and mountains, it all counts. *Terroir* is the land communicating with the food.

Têtoir reflects people and culture. It is in part the accumulated skill sets of creative people, but also the power of a locus, for whatever reason, to attract and breed artisans and artists.

Têtoir builds when the know-how and philosophy of making and creating are passed on from one person to the next. It may start with one chef or a single artisan with a powerful idea, or it can be many artists or craftspeople feeding off the same energy. It can start in a kitchen, like Chez Panisse, or with a group of abstract expressionists drinking beer in Greenwich Village. It can be hyperlocal, regional, or even national. New York City has many *têtoirs*— some that are sophisticated, some street smart, but all honed by tremendous competition. Not much besides talent grows here.

On one level, Chicago's *têtoir* is one of electric blues, and New York City's is one of rhythm and blues, bebop, and Tin Pan Alley. And then, when it comes to jazz and blues, New Orleans has its very own, very personal, very nuanced musical *têtoir*. But no place holds more purchase on the provenance of American roots music than Mississippi.

New York is also a fervent locus for fashion and art, as is

Paris, although no one could confuse the two. Berkeley has its own thing, double-boiled from a tradition of free speech and the food revolution begun by Alice Waters.

Hollywood, as a company town, has its own *têtoir*, from the legacy of Sam Goldwyn to members of the Academy and Local 600 — although how many good pictures actually come out of Hollywood is debatable. Where spectacle and high art once ruled, there is now a lot of commodified fluff.

Hollywood is certainly not alone in producing junk. Look around your house. How many things do you own that are truly handmade and that testify to the talent that created them, whether it is a chair, a hairbrush, a bottle of beer, a hammer — like pop songs that are indistinguishable from a million others?

The corporate mentality that peaked in America in the late nineteenth century at the height of the Industrial Revolution was the beginning of a shift away from artisans and their apprentices, from celebrating the virtues of *terroir* and *têtoir*. Along with manufacturing technology came the futurist battle cry of "fast-faster-fastest!" and the greed that tempted business owners to speed up the slow and steady processes of quality and eliminate, wherever possible, the charming inconsistencies of genuine craft. Generations of accumulated *têtoir* suffered as a result, and by the second half of the twentieth century, a dehumanized, mechanized system of manufacturing and mass production replaced much of the world's *têtoir*.

Brooklyn *têtoir* has shifted over the years. Once upon a time it may have been the disco inferno of Tony Manero and *Saturday Night Fever*—more recently, Jay-Z is top cat. But it has always been about who could throw down the best. There is accumulated knowledge here; we know how to sing and dance and defend street corners. Artists flock here. Now Brooklyn is the epicenter of a new hip, as derided and misunderstood as any social movement—but also the Mecca for a new explosion of gastronomy and literature, to name but two of the borough's enormous contributions. There is likely more talent here per square mile than anyplace else on Earth.

Wherever genuine *têtoir* is found—in art or in craft—it must be celebrated. In microbreweries in Portland, slaughterhouses in Kansas City, chess clubs in Boston, footstool factories in Blaine, the professional wrestling brain trust in Stamford, and the techie start-ups in Silicon Valley, *têtoir* is the best of who we are.

CHAPTER 12

Twelve Great American *Têtoirs*

If your culture doesn't like geeks, you are in real trouble.

—*Bill Gates*

1. The American South

Passed down across generations, the kitchen culture of the American South has blossomed into one of our greatest culinary *têtoirs*. Shrimp and grits, fried chicken, blackened fish, collard greens, BBQ, and corn bread (to name but a few totems of southern cuisine) can be found in some form all across the southeastern United States, prepared within a myriad of traditions born of different races and economic means, by folks who all consider themselves southerners. And you can bet that each kitchen will lay claim to doing it best, with the kind of collegial competition that has made this great locus of American gastronomy so rich (chronicled impeccably by the Southern Foodways Alliance). The South's slow ethic of food and hospitality (not to mention whiskey, music, and literature) passed down from generation to generation makes it an unimpeachable source of great American *têtoir*.

2. American Beer

Knowledge and skills, passed from brewmasters to apprentices in the shadows of shiny silver vats in the hearts of big cities and in small towns, have created an American *têtoir* that few would dispute is the best of its kind in the world.

Perhaps no part of the food movement has grown faster on a national level than that of the microbreweries. In the 1970s you could count the number of breweries that existed in the States on your fingers—and back then only a few imports were available. But within the next few decades more than three thousand new breweries opened their doors, including a few larger independents, which were so successful as to radically influence the quality of beers offered at every American bar and wherever beer is sold.

With few exceptions, making beer is about style and doesn't depend on where it's made, and thus *têtoir* is the correct term to explain the proliferation of the American brewing culture. American brewers are now competitive with (some would say even better than) the traditionally heralded Old World brewmasters.

3. New York City

Sheer population density is the secret: People breed competition, and competition breeds expertise. You name the food category, a *têtoir* for it exists in a New York kitchen—bagels, knishes, smoked fish, cured meats, expertly aged cheese, death-defying sandwiches...it's all here.

The art of the restaurant continues to explode in New York, spinning out of the kitchens of the Meyers and Changs and Feinbergs and Batalis—from old-school Sichuan joints in Queens, to Lucali's pizza and the salad station at Tanoreen in Brooklyn, nowhere else has food culture been refined so well, and become so accessible. Cutting-edge food technology—*sous vide* machines! Immersion circulators!—are pioneering here, as is a slow, back-to-the-garden ethic that has become a national fascination. And it all happens within a few square miles, and in the smallest and most unexpected spaces, often created by people you will never meet.

4. Vermont

It's cold in Vermont—the growing season lasts a fraction as long as it does in the South. But that has not stopped Vermonters from doing an excellent job of adding value to the foods that can be produced there, and then marketing them effectively: "Made in Vermont" is an imprimatur of real value. Companies like Jasper Hill Farm and Cabot Creamery are among the leaders in a cheese revolution that can now compete with the best of Europe—they have literally carved temperature-controlled caves out of mountainsides to age cheese for artisan cheese makers around the state. Meanwhile, Vermonters have mastered, in the sugarhouses that pepper the state, the art of concentrating the sweet liquid that oozes from their maple trees to make what for many is the only acceptable maple syrup.

In Vermont there has always been a strong "buy local" ethic that is the foundation for the state's food *têtoir*. People support small farms and small business; it's a big part of Vermont pride and tradition. Even the way the roads are laid out fosters community: Vermont made a deliberate choice to have only two major north-south interstate highways (and enacted a no-billboards law)—which means that when you have to get from here to there, you have to take the local roads, and small business isn't so easily knocked out in favor of convenience or expediency.

5. The Independent American Fisherman

So large do the American fisherman and the allure of fishing loom in our imaginations that they have created a perfect storm of movies, TV shows, and an entire industry for hobbyists and vacationers looking to drop lines in the water.

Like farmers, ranchers, and hunters, fishermen carry with them legacies and expertise that have been handed down since the first settlers came to America from across the seas. They learned how to read the waters and predict migration routes of animals that they cannot see, a job that only becomes more challenging as stricter environmental regulations limit what they can fish.

Unlike farming, commercial fishing can be a radically dangerous business—commercial fishermen deal with the kind of brutal conditions that no hobbyist could possibly imagine, or even survive: wickedly cold weather and high winds, and the pressure of catching enough fish to make a living in a short fishing season. Through it all, the American fisherman remains one of the most independent and fearless bearers of a grand American *têtoir*.

6. Cocktail Culture

Behind bars there is an incredible *têtoir* being shaken and stirred. The cocktail shaker and martini glass are the universal symbols of civility, culture, and good times, and a uniquely American phenomenon. Cocktails entered the fray of hedonistic gastronomy in large part thanks to Jerry Thomas, often called the father of mixology, a titan of libation who elevated mixing drinks to a high art with his boozy 1862 Baedeker *The Bar-Tender's Guide*. Since then cocktail culture has waxed and waned (and even survived

Prohibition), but what we have witnessed on this side of the new millennium is nothing short of a revolution. Today's mixologist is one part scientist, one part chef, one part historian, and responsible for adding entire new menus to the dining experience, both before and after dinner.

The *têtoir* of the cocktail has led to drinks of astonishing complexity that are time intensive to create, with recipes as varied as any cuisine. They cost as much as or more than an appetizer and deliver pure epiphanies with every nuanced detail—a formulary of drink-specific glassware and hard-as-diamonds ice; a farmers' market's worth of fresh herbs and an apothecary shop's worth of tinctures, handcrafted bitters, and exotic ingredients; not to mention liquor of a specific provenance and unbending quality. No longer confined to America, the art and science of mixology is now gaining a foothold in every civilized country, flowing from the New World to the Old as tomatoes, corn, and tobacco once did, making this *têtoir* an international school of pleasure.

7. Kansas City

Kansas City is the meat capital of the United States. Its *têtoir* is born of the people who work in stockyards and steakhouses. Even as Chicago was celebrated as the "hog butcher to the world," KC, serendipitously located close to the geographical center of the United States, became a hub for getting products, especially agricultural products, to the rest of the country, and built up the infrastructure for meat-packing and trucking.

Outside New York, the strip steak is better known as the Kansas City Strip, and along with Texas, Memphis, and the Carolinas, Kansas City is a world capital of barbecue. Kansas City boasts more than ninety barbecue restaurants in the metropolitan area alone and hosts the world's biggest barbecue contest.

You can find pretty much any kind of meat in Kansas City, including heritage breeds, all cooked low and slow, from beef and pork to mutton and turkeys—but what we love best is KC's famous burnt ends, the charred edges of brisket. Call it nose to tail or just good eats, in Kansas City they know better than to let those carbon-blackened jewels go to waste.

8. The Amish

Amish people can be found in many places, but primarily in southeastern Pennsylvania, Maryland, West Virginia, North Carolina, and Ohio. Agriculture is at the center of Amish life and, with rare exceptions, every member of every Amish household is somehow involved with the farm and food production.

While some of the *terroirs* the Amish till are certainly special, it is the accumulated skill sets and agricultural

know-how passed on from one generation to the next—
the *têtoir*—that are the most remarkable. I'm fortunate to
have befriended an Amish family in Ohio, a relationship
that has lasted for twenty-five years, and I have experienced
firsthand an inspirational *têtoir* of self-sufficiency and business savvy that extends from running and building farms
to embracing organic techniques for their dairies that
would make any American stand up and applaud. Their
hard work is closely connected to their belief in God—and
their faith has led to the creation of the strongest agricultural group in the United States.

9. Portland

As comedian Fred Armisen riffs in his charming television series *Portlandia*, the dream of the 1890s is alive in
Portland—which naturally makes it a favorite destination
for the old men who wrote THE CARNIVORE'S MANIFESTO.
This is a city that is properly obsessed with sustainability
and artisanal skills, and with sharing the knowledge and
joy with anyone who will listen. That Portland is America's most literate city makes us love it all the more. There
is something about this jewel of the Pacific Northwest
that attracts a thinking and capable populace who create
plenty to occupy their hands and minds on numerous
rainy days.

Portland's coffee culture is legend, and its part in the
American microbrew revolution earned it the nickname

Beervana. Portland has more than sixty breweries—more than any other city in the world—a *têtoir* supported by the local agriculture, namely the famed two-row barley, several dozen varieties of hops, and water from the Bull Run watershed.

When it comes to restaurants, Portland can go toe-to-toe with any larger city and is surely among the three or four best cities in the country to sit down and eat in, but it is also a Mecca of street food: Portland is at the vanguard of the food cart uprising as well.

As in Brooklyn, a confluence of location and culture has created a nexus of like-minded people in Portland who are spawning a new wave of wickedly diverse businesses and hobbies, from bakeries to backyard chicken coops and taxidermy shops—but with a population of only about six hundred thousand, there is likely more good, sustainable, artisanal, slow food per capita in Portland than anyplace in America.

10. New Orleans

No city in America has captured our romantic imagination more than the Crescent City, New Orleans, Louisiana. As notorious for its secret history of voodoo rituals as it is famous for being the birthplace of jazz, New Orleans continues to astound with an indigenous culture unlike any in the United States. And no matter if it is Mardi Gras or JazzFest, you can bet there will be food involved.

In a world that has been so hyperglobalized that you

can seemingly get any sort of cuisine without leaving home, New Orleans remains alone in that only a trip to the city itself can offer the rewards of genuine Creole food (and the unapologetic pleasure-to-the-point-of-vice with which it is consumed). Many have tried to re-create the true magic of gumbo and jambalaya in other locales but lack the *têtoir* to compete with the real thing.

New Orleans cuisine is the culinary equivalent of jazz, with influences seeping in from Africa and Cuba to spice up the local flavor. Present, too, are notes of Italian cooking (try the muffuletta, a sandwich laid thick with Italian cold cuts and New Orleans proprietary olive salad), and of course, the bounty of the Gulf: oysters and shrimp, often fried and served on po'boy sandwiches, not to mention the nearly mythical Louisiana crawfish. And no discussion of New Orleans is complete without mention of rice and beans, pralines, beignets, and café au lait made with chicory, or alligator pie. This is a city fiercely proud and protective of its traditions and legacy, and even while new restaurants open up that reflect a modern slant on local cuisine, the local *têtoir* is ever present. The citizens of New Orleans would not have it any other way.

11. Berkeley

From the free speech and antiwar movements of the 1960s and moving forward, Berkeley's *têtoir* is one steeped in the fight for fairness and justice. This East Bay city has been a hot spot for a strain of progressive thinking that has taken over the American counterculture at large—few places are so proud of being an instigator on the American stage or so united and vocal in the belief that everyone's voice should be heard.

In 1964 UC Berkeley students fought for the right to use campus facilities for political debate and for the dissemination of political literature, a First Amendment victory that remains at the root of this city's spirit.

In 1971, four years before the fall of Saigon, Alice Waters changed the way we look at food—her Chez Panisse at 1517 Shattuck Avenue is credited as the epicenter of the organic food revolution. Later, her group started the most important public school farm-and-garden program in the nation, the Edible Schoolyard. The worker-owned-and-operated Cheese Board Collective, right across the street from Chez Panisse, is a powerful example of the democratic spirit of Berkeley, as are the hundreds of other nearby small businesses and co-ops that bring power to the people. Berkeley continues to be a lightning rod for creatives and revolutionaries, a beacon for positive politics and enlightenment.

12. Marijuana

Marijuana has a noble and colorful history, from the sunbaked *terroir* of Mexico to the enlightened *têtoir* of

California, where that wonderful strain of hippies-cum-scientists began using their powers for good.

America has always been a country that loves its "muggles," as Louis Armstrong liked to call it. Since the 1920s we've seen movies, magazines, comedy records, and musicians—from Cab Calloway to Willie Nelson to Snoop Dogg—celebrating the herb, and a constant wave of innovative stoner paraphernalia, from acrylic bongs to Frisbees retrofitted with joint-holding gimmicks for stoners to flip to each other at rock concerts. The last fifty years or so, however, have seen the status of cannabis raised from party favor to symbol of protest and libertarianism to legitimate medicine. And now, finally, that the movement to legalize recreational use is beginning to take hold, we are entering the golden age of marijuana.

Marijuana is botany at its apex, all about strains and the subtle differences among plants and methods of cultivation, curing, and consumption. Witness the great wave of beautiful, hand-blown glassware and high-tech vaporizers that have become the standard over the last decade, not to mention cannabis-infused candies, oils, and high-end baked goods. It is a *têtoir* of psychotropic agri-connoisseurship— written reviews of a previously unimaginable sophistication for strains like Purple Blueberry and Strawberry Cough have approached viniculture in developing a proprietary vocabulary to explain the unexplainable.

Marijuana growers are a perfect example of a culture of

shared information and experience. They are the vibrant pioneers of a new type of agriculture, riding an unprecedented crest of opportunity: Large-scale investors are looking to turn marijuana into America's greatest *legitimate* cash crop.

CHAPTER 13

Give the People What They Want

If you are what you eat, then you're fast, cheap, and easy.

—*Deborah Madison*

A Value Meal at McDonald's costs about six bucks, and that includes the price of deforesting South America, running a cruel corporate farming system, and confusing your bloodstream with undue amounts of salt, sugar, and fat. Over at the Meatball Shop in Williamsburg, Brooklyn, eight bucks will get you two gorgeous meatballs made from heritage pork raised on a pasture with nary an antibiotic within screaming range, and they come with a healthy and delicious side vegetable and some wonderful bread.

If more joints like the Meatball Shop opened around America—fast-food style, but slow-food sourced—it would have a massive impact on America's sustainable farming culture, as well as our national health crisis. Chipotle is paving the way, but there is room for so much more.

Competing with fast food is not as hard as you might think: The average steer produces only about five hundred eight-ounce burgers, if you grind the whole thing. A tiny three-by-three-foot grill in a busy location could easily burn through more than three hundred chemical-free, grass-fed cattle a year—nose to tail—supporting an entire network of sustainable farms while delivering great food, fast.

The big fast-food peddlers will never do it right. They have no responsibility to anyone or anything other than the short-term bottom line. They have no ethical imperative, no vision for a healthy country. Their "wraps" and salads are nothing more than a stalking horse, a public relations gimmick.

But there isn't a competent chef in America who couldn't move the dial in the right direction, toward providing slow food, fast—many of them are already doing it on their menus with thoughtful pork buns and a thousand varieties of quality meat on a stick. Now it's time to take that kind of sustainable food out of the finer restaurants and into gas stations and convenience stores. And there isn't an independent farmer who wouldn't leap at the chance to participate.

For the sustainable food movement to make an impact on America's most unhealthy eating habits, we are going to have to play the game of convenience and infiltrate the territory traditionally staked out by McDonald's, Burger King, Taco

Bell, and their ilk—inner cities, suburbs, Midtown Manhattan, shopping malls, airports, and highways, wherever people need to eat quickly and inexpensively. The time has come for a new wave of burger-flipping agri-preneurs to prosper while the old model of fast food fades fast on the wrong side of history!

CHAPTER 14

Hello, I Am a Pig

Homer: Are you saying you're never going to eat
   any animal again? What about bacon?
Lisa: No.
Homer: Ham?
Lisa: No.
Homer: Pork chops?
Lisa: Dad, those all come from the same animal.
Homer: Heh heh heh. Ooh, yeah, right, Lisa. A
   wonderful, magical animal.
   —The Simpsons

Hello, I am a pig.

We are a noble race that has produced heroes, rapscallions, and celebrities, like Piglet, Porky, and Miss Piggy, who has even been mentioned as a possible presidential candidate! Just look at England's most celebrated pig, the

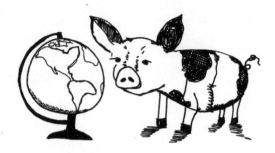

Empress of Blandings, Lord Emsworth's prizewinning sow, and the wonderful stories she inspired, not to mention television's favorite porker, Arnold Ziffel! And can you think of a greater movie star than Babe?

I was first domesticated over ten thousand years ago in a country you call China, and there are now about 900 million of my kind in the world. Wherever I have existed, humans have done well. My domesticated brethren are fertile year-round, offering a reliable source of food. I was the primary source of meat for middle Stone Age peoples. Cro-Magnons drew pictures of my kind on the walls of Altamira more than fifteen thousand years ago.

I was brought to North America by the Vikings, Columbus, Cortés, and de Soto. I settled with you in Jamestown, and the Pilgrims brought me to Massachusetts. I was a principal source of protein for troops in your Revolutionary War.

I am closer than any livestock to a dog in intelligence

and trainability. My kind are meant to scavenge and forage. I used to roam free on city streets, keeping them clean. I find truffles a foot under the soil—my nose is more powerful and discerning than the Eagles, Fleetwood Mac, and Aerosmith at the peak of their snorting powers!

I love to root. In the past I prepared fields for crops and I cleared forested land. I helped your kind build resistance to diseases like influenza, flu, and pertussis. I am a symbol of such strength and nobility that you make coin banks in my image.

But today factory farms have violated the sacred relationship I have developed with you over millennia. Of the 90 million of my kind in the US, almost every one of us is raised in overcrowded barns and tiny pens, leaving us no outlet for our curiosity. No chance to fulfill our God-given natural instincts. This has made us meaner to you, and to each other.

Today most breeds of pigs are the product of corporately concocted genetics, designed in a laboratory to grow too fast and yield unnaturally lean meat. Because of this, we have become weak and prone to illness, and now we need medicine in our food. Dozens of heritage breeds are on the brink of extinction. The chance that my kind will ever again become the strong, proud animal it once was wanes with each sick harvest.

But there is hope. Our light continues to flicker on family farms that dot the surroundings of your farmers' markets and in places like Kansas, where rare and heritage breed associations honor us. Please support us. Lay claim to our future by laying off the industrial bacon and the factory-farmed hams.

We live for you. Show a little respect.

CHAPTER 15

Take My Ham, Please

It's not easy being green.

—*Kermit the Frog*

Slow Food founder Carlo Petrini once called for the "formation of a universal movement in defense of microbes." Talk about standing up for the little guy!

What Carlo was getting at is the hell-bent American mission to destroy all known germs and bacteria. In the United States, we sanitize everything to the point where we are reducing our immune systems to vestigial ghosts. Count on it, this is one phobia that is going to come back and bite us in the ass. If we pretend to live in a bubble, we'll end up like the boy in the bubble, cut off from the ability to resist even the most mundane of germs.

Our germ phobia is also hurting American artisans' ability to create a great food culture that competes with that of Europe, perhaps best represented by the big ol' legs of ham that sit on the bars or hang from the ceilings in pretty much every restaurant or hole-in-the-wall bar in Italy and Spain.

Our friends at Salumeria Biellese in New York cure meats that are very similar to those in the Old Country — but they had to pay hundreds of thousands of dollars to run a myriad of tests at Cornell University to prove to the United States Department of Agriculture and local health departments that there are no harmful levels of bacteria on meats cured using their Old World methods. Now Biellese produces delicious meats for wholesale and retail throughout the country, but it cost them a bundle to break down that wall. Most artisans don't have those resources and have no choice but to obey the hyperhygienic guidelines of health agencies that are simply aren't interested in establishing a new set of rules for traditional curing.

The irony is that while the government is up in arms over someone's salami, it continues to shift upward the allowable amount of toxins in our air and water and still rate them clean, another favor to Big Ag and any business that needs a little leeway when it comes to dumping its toxic waste. The government also allows for the treatment of beef trimmings with ammonia to create what is now called pink slime. It makes zero sense.

The USDA and local health departments need to grow with the artisan food movement and support research on behalf of small producers in restaurants and test kitchens who rely on the nuance of taste to differentiate their superior products from commodity counterparts. Producing great food should not be the domain solely of companies that can pay for testing.

It's easy for the USDA to just say no—they have no real incentive to work for small producers. The USDA has only about eight thousand inspectors, who are already overworked, and they don't even follow food through the entire production process—they just sort of show up at the end and whip out their petri dishes and biogadgets. They like to look at one slice of salami while ignoring the pig's life, what it ate, how healthy it was, and how it came to be a tasty salami in the first place. This is an example of where we need more government and not less. We need more boots on the ground following our food from farm to truck and beyond.

Our health and safety agencies need new standards for artisans and responsible chefs, and for small-farm products that come from a system free of chemicals and bad genetics.

For instance, currently the USDA-recommended internal temperatures for cooking meats are still ten to fifteen degrees higher than they need to be for quality food to be safe to eat, effectively obliterating any taste in good meat—a service to commodity producers whose mediocre products taste "better" when the actual taste is cooked out. It's too bad so many people still live in fear and feel they need to nuke their heritage chops to the point of gastronomic tragedy. At least two recommended temperatures should be promoted—one for fast food and one for slow food.

Perhaps we should also consider an "eat at your own risk" label. Even with a warning label, I would trust the charcuterie station at Gramercy Tavern more than any food from Smithfield.

The USDA and local departments of health are rightfully on the lookout for bacteria that can be harmful to humans. And they have done a great job of protecting Americans from the dangers of these enemies. But we would all benefit if they became more of a yes organization, attuned to researching the techniques behind century-old traditions.

In other words, take my ham, please.

CHAPTER 16

You Can't Avoid Processed Food

My dear, here we must run as fast as we can, just to
stay in place. And if you wish to go anywhere you
must run twice as fast as that.

    —*Lewis Carroll,* Alice's Adventures in
Wonderland

Forget your hippie dream of eating 100 percent organic,
because it's not going to happen. Let's be honest: It is just
not doable if you are living any kind of real life.

Confined turkeys are a reality. It makes me sick. I have
dedicated myself to changing that, but what am I going to
do, I mean on a day-to-day, real-life, don't-confuse-my-
dreams-with-reality basis? I confess, I eat a turkey sandwich
from a deli or a diner once in a while, and I know that turkey did not lead a good life. It sucks, but I work in New
York, and every now and again I welcome a club sandwich

into my world. Same with the bacon I eat with my eggs in any greasy spoon anywhere in America—it is industrial-farmed commodity pork, everything I fight against.

Eat only plants? Don't eat foods with more than three ingredients? Never eat Snickers bars? You have to make your own rules, principles that you can live by, with an eye on moving the dial toward the healthy and humane. The best I can tell, even the most thoughtful eater is going to be eating commodity food a quarter of the time—and just to get there you have to be industrious and focused almost nonstop. Even hard-cores like Alice Waters accept nonorganic options, as long as the producers are moving in the right direction. Be realistic. One hundred percent organic? All local, fresh, and unprocessed? That's a nice idea, but ultimately it's crazy talk. Unabomber shit.

As I'm writing this, I'm eating a fantastic slab of Brooklyn pizza—white processed flour, tomato sauce hijacked by high-fructose corn syrup, pepperoni that comes from God knows where, and I love it. Maybe cereal that changes the color of the milk isn't good for you, but neither is artisanal vodka, organic weed, or cocaine from the mountains of Peru farmed by grass-fed llamas; but honestly, they all have their place.

Mark Twain used to tell a story. He was with a woman who was on her deathbed, and he wanted to lighten her load.

"Madam," he said, "do you smoke? Do you drink?"

"No."

"Do you gamble?"

"No."

"Do you have any vices at all?"

"No," she said.

"Just as I thought—a sinking ship with no ballast to throw overboard!"

CHAPTER 17

Eat an Endangered Species

When the last individual of a race of living things
breathes no more, another Heaven and another
Earth must pass before such a one can be again.
— *William Beebe*

I sometimes ask people what the main difference is between
the Red Wattle pig and the Bengali tiger, and the answer is
that there are more Bengali tigers in the world than there
are Red Wattle breeding pigs. Red Wattles are also delicious, and legal to eat.

There are dozens of varieties of chickens, ducks, geese,
pigs, and cows on the endangered species list as a direct
consequence of industrial farming and food conglomerates. Promoting biodiversity is not on the agenda for the
Industrial Food Complex, which has no incentive except to
churn out only one breed of beast (made from genetic engineering and Dr. Moreau–like biowrenching), the one that

produces the largest amount of white meat in the shortest time. The corporate mantra is *more food faster*—cheap food at any cost!—until no market exists for anything else, no matter how severe the consequences or how small an investment it would take to change course.

Because these are livestock and poultry, we don't see them in the same way as we do more exotic animals that people pay money to see in zoos. But just as there are many kinds of dogs and cats in the world, so are there many varieties of pigs, goats, sheep, and cows.* No one's

---

* Just to give you an idea of how great the diversity of wonderfully delicious animals is, here's a list of noncommodity, heritage, and rare breeds from *The Encyclopedia of Historic and Endangered Livestock and Poultry Breeds*, by Janet Vorwald Dohner. GOATS: English, Bagot, Golden Guernsey, San Clemente, Spanish, Tennessee Fainting, Myotonic, Wooden Leg, Nigerian Dwarf, Oberhasli, Isle of Man, Irish, Scottish, Hawaiian, Arapawa, Saturna Island, Mona Island. SHEEP: Soay, Shetland, North Ronaldsay, Hebridean, Manx Loaghtan, Jacob, Boreray, Castlemilk Moorit, Welsh Mountain, Black Welsh Mountain, Torddu, Torwen, Balwen, Hill Radnor, Lleyn, Portland, Dorset Horn, Wiltshire Horn, Whitefaced Woodland, Lincoln, Teeswater, Wensleydale, Leicester Longwool, Cotswold, Galway, Devon, Cornwall Longwool, White Face and Greyface Dartmoors, Ryeland, Herdwick, Southdown, Oxford Down, Dorset Down, Shropshire, Norfolk Horn, Clun Forest, Kerry Hill, Llanwenog, Navajo-Churro, Santa Cruz, Gulf Coast Native, Newfoundland Local, Hog Island, Tunis, Delaine Merino, Caribbean Hair, Boricua, Barbados Blackbelly, Virgin Island White, St. Croix, Katahdin, Karakul, Feral Hawaiian. PIGS: Tamworth, British Saddleback, Gloucestershire Old Spot, British Lop, Berkshire, Middle White, Large Black, Oxford Sandy and Black, Ossabaw Island, Guinea, Poland China, American Mulefoot, Red Wattle, Choctaw, Hereford. CATTLE: White Park, American White Park, Vaynol, Chillingham, Highland, Kerry, Dexter, English Longhorn, Ayrshire, Shetland, Red Poll, Irish Moiled, Galloway, White Galloway, Belted Galloway, British White, Devon, Milking Devon, Gloucester,

saying to fricassee a Komodo dragon or cacciatore an American bald eagle, but you should definitely think about roasting a Gloucestershire Old Spot pig, or grilling a Tunis lamb.

It seems like laughing in the face of God to willfully crush biodiversity for the sake of overdeveloping one breed for profit. How haughty do you have to be to drive into extinction a noble breed that had been raised by generations of family farms, that had its own traits and taste and look and purpose—like the Red Wattle, which populated the yards of New Orleans throughout the eighteenth and nineteenth centuries?

We've already seen the food chain polluted with swine flu and bird flu and mad cow disease—how remote a possibility do you think it is that Thanksgiving could get canceled some year because of one ambitious germ that affects one breed but not another (heritage breeds of poultry have proved to survive bird flu better than their commodity cousins)? The Irish potato famine wouldn't have happened if the Irish hadn't been reliant on just one breed of potato. If they had had more diversity they would have been left with plenty of crops.

Forty-five million turkeys will be sold this Thanksgiving, so industrial turkey producers who only raise one or

---

Shorthorn, Beef Shorthorn, Northern Dairy Shorthorn, Whitebred Shorthorn, Lincoln Red, Milking Shorthorn, Guernsey, Florida Cracker and Pineywoods, Texas Longhorn, Canadienne, Dutch Belt, Lineback, Randall Blue Lineback, Ankole Watusi.

two varieties aren't doing so badly for themselves. But trust me when I tell you they are living in a very tenuous place. Because of the reliance on a single strain of the Broad Breasted White, entire flocks are one novel pathogen away from being wiped off the American dinner table. It would be like *The Andromeda Strain,* or *Twelve Monkeys,* or *The Hot Zone*—but for turkeys. But then, maybe you'd like to spend Thanksgiving in a museum showing your kids what a turkey used to look like.

Imagine that the family of the famed French professional wrestler and gastronome André the Giant has a small herd of heirloom cattle in the French Alps, bred especially for that specific altitude, with a unique taste that comes from grazing on that particular Alpine grass, and coddled in drunken French (and occasionally Swiss). The community builds its local gastronomy around the herd, and a few connoisseurs come in search of it, but mostly André's family sends meat to the local bistro for the few people left who have grown up enjoying this unique pleasure. Eventually the old family farm will be shut out by a system that is gamed against local heritage and skewed toward commodity. Mr. and Mrs. André the Giant get old and die, and there is almost no incentive for anyone to continue raising this breed of cattle. Why? It takes too much work, it's too expensive, and the market for quality meat is dwindling because most people are happy eating whatever is put in front of them. These cows now are going the way of the dodo bird. Gone. From the earth. Forever.

Breeding and slaughtering these animals is part of the responsible stewardship of the planet. It may be counterintuitive—some kind of inverse Darwinism that contradicts that whole survival-of-the-fittest thing—but to save them, we've got to eat them.

CHAPTER 18

Slow Business, Part I: Meet Me in the Middle

Corporation: An ingenious device for obtaining individual profit without individual responsibility.

—*Ambrose Bierce*

Supermarket chains may think they have little choice but to be engines of efficiency, but along with their low prices comes a high cost—they are part of what I consider a national blight: the systematic extinction of the empowered middle manager.

Once upon a time, grocery stores bought food from vendors who would show up with the day's haul—a truckload of fresh produce, fish, bread, or meat. The actual grocers themselves made the buying decisions—they were the boots on the ground, and they were the product of a wonderful *têtoir*. They knew fresh food and good deals and what their community wanted and needed. Everyone in the local economy benefitted, from the farmers to the customers. There was bonhomie all around, and good food-chain feng shui! But right now I am betting there is no one at your local supermarket who could pull the trigger and write a check for a bushel of fresh peaches from a local farmer.

Can you imagine if independent local farmers could bring their produce directly to the store after a day manning their market stand, instead of having to drive it back home and store it, maybe even throw it out? The potential to transform local agriculture would be amazing—"Hey, I know this guy! His lettuce is the best! What beautiful beets! I love his turnips! And those strawberries? Once-in-a-lifetime sweet! And he is going to give me a good price, and our customers are going to be very happy."

Corporate supermarket chains and big-box stores are managed from the top down. No longer are the workers on the floor in your neighborhood market in touch with the source of your food. Nor are they empowered to make any decisions. Mostly they just stock shelves. All the decisions are made remotely, and as a system, the chains can only buy from a limited number of approved vendors, which unfortunately won't include a lot of small, local independent farms.

This isn't much better than old-school Taylorism, the paranoid system of so-called scientific management and synthesized workflow that treats workers like drones, incapable of understanding anything much beyond brainless piecework. In this model, workers are rigidly controlled—they are cogs in the machine with little or no hope of advancing to a position that will help them tap into their full potential.

This ruthless worldview was first formalized by Frederick Winslow Taylor in tracts like *A Piece-Rate System* (1895), *Shop Management* (1903), and *The Principles of Scientific Management* (1911), and has had the dismal effect of alienating and de-skilling the American work force.

Henry Ford and Walt Disney were pioneers of Taylorism, robbing potential from the very people who made them so rich. Mentoring workers, they argued, just took too much time. At the Ford Motor Company, this conveyor-belt mentality meant that during the course of a day, a month, a year, one worker might only do one task, over and over again. At Disney, assembly-line designers were forced to draw one detail of a cartoon endlessly rather than learn the entire process of design, like painting Mickey's gloves white, over and over and over again. It was mind-numbing work, and although it may have taken more finesse to draw than to drop a windshield into a car body, and it might have contributed to the genius of, say, *Fantasia,* in no way was the cat who painted the mouse's hands ever going to become a great artist unless he could somehow punch through the wall of corporate efficiency. That sort of drive and ambition was frowned upon. It wasn't good for business.

Banks were once the strongest bastions of middle management—men and women at your savings and loan were authorized to make loans and mortgages, extend lines of credit, and foster growth. Now try finding someone at a bank who can make a decision for you, or help in any meaningful way.

Recently I was the victim of identity theft. I got socked for all sorts of stuff someone else was charging to my account. Naturally, I alerted the bank as soon as possible, and what did they do for me? They canceled my credit until they could investigate further. They were in no hurry to help me, they just shut it all down. The guy I talked to, a junior executive, said, "I know, buddy, it sucks. Wish I could help you. But I can't." Corporate mentality assumes the worst of people.

Many respectable jobs have been stripped of their dignity and purpose. In the food world, middle managers should be trusted and encouraged to facilitate local relationships and expand the network of approved vendors. A good market is one that sources from the best vendors, not just one industrial hub. You can't expect a CEO and his board to know where the best pork comes from, nor the apples with which to serve it.

CHAPTER 19

Don't Make Ketchup

Health food may be good for the conscience but
Oreos taste a hell of a lot better.
— *Robert Redford*

Marion Cunningham, James Beard's former assistant who
went on to be an inspirational food writer, was famous for
saying that Hellmann's is the best mayo in the world. Mark
Ladner, executive chef at Del Posto — the only Italian restaurant ever to get four stars from the *New York Times* —
swears that Gulden's is the finest mustard ever made. When
you want Worcestershire sauce, do any two names mean
more than Lea & Perrins? And what kind of ass must you
be to think you could possibly make an egg cream with
anything other than Fox's U-Bet syrup from Brooklyn?

Artisanal is awesome, but no matter what you make,
you always have to compete with the best, or else why

would people want it? And especially when it comes to no-brainer staples, why are you even wasting your time?

How many restaurants have I been to that presume to make a better ketchup than Heinz, only to serve up ersatz simulacra of same? First, where are these chefs getting the tomatoes in the middle of winter? And even if it were August, and even if you lived in the heart of the Garden State, is that really what you want to be doing with your gorgeous produce—making ketchup? But the truth—metaphysical, existential, and for real—is that a bottle of Heinz is a tribute to American cuisine, not a commodified insult.

Small-batch doesn't necessarily mean good, nor does coming from a small farm guarantee amazing taste. There is a lot of mediocre stuff being made, everywhere, often in the name of improving on an existing commodity product.

Let's be real: Tabasco is what your oyster wants. There is room for a hundred hot sauces, but there is only one for your oyster and it's from Avery Island in Louisiana. The ingredients are vinegar, red peppers, and salt. What manner of culinary alchemy is going to top that?

We've suffered enough as a people without self-righteous do-it-yourselfers trying to re-create Coca-Cola. You put this stuff in your mouth. It has to be good.

CHAPTER 20

Nose to Tail: Let's Grind

The way you cut your meat reflects the way you
live.

—*Confucius*

Ground meat is the salvation of the American independent
farmer. If you want to get serious about being a part of the
sustainable food movement, now is the time to eat a burger.
Or a meatball. Or make a ragù, at least! Everyone benefits,
from the farmer who gets paid more per animal if his ground
meat gets sold at a fair price, to the small-slaughterhouse
owner who needs more business, and finally to the consumer
who gets the lowest per-portion cost in the meat world.

Forget whatever you read in some precious foodie magazine about nose-to-tail cooking. If the new farm movement is going to take off—including more grass-fed cattle
operations and significant growth in the domestic lamb
and goat trade—it will be a lot easier and better for

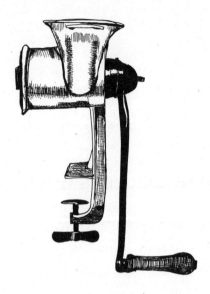

everyone involved if the trend is toward grinding the most meat possible.

I can respect someone for boiling a cow's head, but that's not an equation for launching a fast-food alternative. People call Heritage Foods all the time and say, "Hey, I really want to help your movement, can you send me twenty pig faces so we can make pig's head terrine?" Oy vey — what would really help is if they wanted a hundred pounds of 60-percent-lean trim to make sausages.

On an average eight-hundred-pound steer on the rail, I've seen between 20 and 80 percent turned into ground. It's very simple: The more meat that is ground, the fewer pieces the farmer needs to worry about selling. There are a hundred ways to cut up a cow, but how great is it when the farmer only has to worry about a few? Lower cuts — like the beef rounds, which can weigh up to eighty pounds per animal—just aren't that popular as pieces, whether on the butcher counter or on the menu.

My friends who started the restaurant Farm 255 in Athens, Georgia, are a model when it comes to the potential of *true* nose-to-tail cooking. They had a farm, Moonshine Meats, that supplied their restaurant with 100 percent grass-fed beef. As the restaurant grew, other neighboring farms got on board to help meet demand. More farms meant more animals, and more complications in getting rid of the myriad of cuts, so they had the vision to open another restaurant, Farm Burger, which became immediately popular by selling terrific ground meat as burgers.

Now there are three Farm Burger locales—practically a chain!—and more farmers are signing on every day, grinding up to 80 percent of each animal, a tremendous achievement. And they are able to sell the few remaining premium cuts—the rib eye, the strip, and the tenderloin—at a lower price, and never get stuck with inventory. Everything moves. New farms are created and old ones are empowered with new business. And the Slow Food movement keeps marching on.

This all goes for lamb as well—if domestic lamb is ever going to become a growth market (instead of our importing it from New Zealand), we need to eat more ground lamb. And it also goes for goats, a great protein source and a potential profit center for independent family farmers because goats are low-maintenance livestock. When it comes to making chili or an unexpected ragù, you might want to think about lamb or goat.

Poultry is a bit different. It should always be the goal of the independent poultry farmer to sell whole birds and not deal with leftover parts. But any bird that is not completely Grade A from top to bottom—because of a bruise on the wing or a discoloration or whatever—that bird has to be cut up and sold in pieces. A turkey farmer has no choice but to grind about 10 percent of his flock every year around Thanksgiving. So the more ground turkey—or chicken—we consume, the easier it is for independent farmers to know that they only have one thing to move besides the whole bird.

No one has set a higher bar for the potential of grinding meat creatively than the storied New York meat distributor Pat LaFrieda. LaFrieda—actually there are two of them, Sr. and Jr.—is king of special textures and the refined taste of the grind. The two have become rock stars based on their talents for mixing different cuts from different livestock into ground meat and reminding the world that there is a lot more to making a great burger than beef chuck. Their mix is the secret of the Shake Shack burgers' buttery taste, and their other mash-ups make the magic between some of New York's best-loved buns, including those of Minetta Tavern, Union Square Cafe, and the Spotted Pig.

You can even grind your own meat and bring the movement right into your home. Why not? Become an expert mixologist! A good grinder will bring new life to any meat you have left over—throw that uncooked flank in there with the sirloin you never got around to eating and you will be a hero to your family, a baron of the barbecue, hailed as a Burger Meister throughout the land! Your chilis, pasta sauces, and stuffed peppers will be celebrated as conquering heroes! But remember, as everyone who has seen *Goodfellas* knows, when you are making a meatball (in prison or otherwise), "You gotta have the pork. That's the flavor."

CHAPTER 21

Not-So-Candid Camera

Were the walls of our meat industry to become
transparent, literally or even figuratively, we
would not long continue to raise, kill, and eat animals the way we do.

—*Michael Pollan*, The Omnivore's Dilemma

Dear Industrial Food Complex,

*There are cameras everywhere in America. There is
hardly a square meter in any big city that is not under sur-
veillance in one way or another, and despite the invasion of
privacy, the populace applauds this sort of Big Brother
approach to security. So why is it that concentrated feeding
operations and slaughterhouses, where ten billion animals
are processed every year, are the last places on Earth where
cameras are not allowed? We have more cameras in outer
space!*

Until you allow a responsible third-party arbiter to monitor your key points of production, you are presumed guilty of animal abuse and cruelty.

It is the fundamental right of all Americans to know exactly what they are putting in their mouths.

Sincerely,

THE CARNIVORE'S MANIFESTO

CHAPTER 22

Sleep with Your Butcher. And Maybe Your Bartender.

If more of us valued food and cheer and song above
hoarded gold, it would be a merrier world.

—*J. R. R. Tolkien*

There is no better way to maintain your place on top of the
food chain than by having an intimate relationship with
your butcher—or, for that matter, your produce guy, your
bread baker, your cheesemonger, maybe a spice gal, and a
local pastry prodigy.

In fact, can you name five local food shops with which
you do business? If you can't, then you are probably not
part of the sustainable food movement. These relationships
are intimate and nurturing.

Take the butcher. He or she is, after all, the gatekeeper,
the last stop between you and the meat you put in your

mouth. And when you think about it in those terms, do we have to explain just how important a relationship that is?

Think about just how much can go wrong during a casual hookup with a butcher you hardly know: When you are eating his ground meat, are you sure you know what you're getting? Does the meat come from some sad and horrible place?

Perhaps his technique leaves something to be desired. Perhaps he doesn't know just where your pleasure center lies—or doesn't care. Maybe his wife likes her pot roast dry and well done and it has made him bitter. Maybe he has you confused with Mrs. Jones down the street who shops only on price point, or Frannie from Scarsdale who has to be convinced that there is Angus something or other in her burger meat, even though she couldn't tell a Big Mac from the burger at the Four Seasons if her fur coat depended on it.

Just the way you choose a life partner, choose your butcher wisely. And then get close to him or her and learn the secrets. Don't be afraid of intimacy. Shake that fear of commitment! Be emotionally available to your butcher, because he (or she) has needs, too. He lives to please you with his bone-in strip and his immaculate flank steak, and if he is a good butcher, he'll have great ideas how about how to cook them, things you might not have thought of: Flank Steak Mephisto Style or the proper way to do Pork Chops Murphy.

He knows where the meat comes from, he can steer

you away from inferior choices and toward the best product. Be his confidant and never again will you hear "I've got some lovely lamb chops" when all he wants to do is dump tired inventory.

And after you've been with him a few times, he will know your taste. No more fumbling foreplay with the London broil, and even the simplest assignation can turn into unexpected pleasure.

Last Saturday night when I was looking for a skirt steak to throw on the grill for a casual Sunday-afternoon barbecue just for two, my butcher Emile motioned with her finger and asked me to help her out. "I've got two nice shell steaks here, much better than the skirt. They're gorgeous, and I'd love to get rid of them so I can start in on a fresh cow Tuesday—do me a favor, take them home, you won't be sorry."

It was hard to say no to the lady who double-cuts my pork chops without having to ask (they always look like something straight out of a Dr. Seuss book), and sure enough, the difference in choice seemed to evaporate when I got home and discovered that some particularly toothsome Basque sausages had leapt into my bag, and that the shell steaks were extraordinary. Just as in love, openness and willingness to take chances are rewarded in those magical little ways that make a relationship special.

And when you are done romancing the butcher in the morning, you should think about getting together with the cheesemonger, who will make the wine you buy from your independent wine merchant so much more worthwhile, and then, when cocktail hour strikes, your favorite local bartender.

Don't be a one-stop shopper. You should consider patronizing a local florist, a baker, a pastry shop, a fishmonger, a vegetable stand, a gelato truck. Spreading your dollars over many small businesses and encouraging independence is a key to the sustainable food movement. Hell, I married my cheesemonger and life has never been better.

But my relationship with my bartender is romantic, too. He just looks at me and knows what I need. When I need an energy boost, he knows to mix me the perfect Negroni, just the way I like it, and when he is onto a new concoction, he shares it with me, he tests his newfound mixology on me and my pals — friends-and-family style — and we all leave soused and just a little bit wiser.

This isn't the model for a free-love utopia, this is about beating down the market forces of commodity and building a community. I've said it before — what could be more intimate than putting something in your mouth, whether it's pink like a veal chop, or sweet and wet like a domestic vermouth. Be loyal to those who give you the real love, and you will enter a dome of locally sourced pleasure that Coleridge could only have dreamed of.

CHAPTER 23

And the Truck Driver Shall Inherit the Earth

When somebody blazes a path to a highway that
never end, you should appreciate 'em some.

— *Brownie McGhee*

There is a threatened culture on the American roadways,
one that affects us all: the culture of the truck driver, the
man or woman on whose back this country runs.

At the top of the food world we see celebrity chefs and
fabulous restaurateurs, sexy bartenders, toothy television
personalities, glib food writers, and hopefully farmers and
butchers, too. But the American truck driver is a hero in all
of this, so please, let's take a moment to sing the truck driver's song.

Once upon a time that anthem was Dave Dudley's
smash "Six Days on the Road." Later, "Convoy," a 1970s

novelty tune that rode on the fad of CB culture, was a number-one smash: "Pig Pen, this here's Rubber Duck and I'm about to put the hammer down!" CB lingo is the Yiddish of the open road.

The seventies also saw a spate of movies that romanticized truckers as outlaws, from the classic *White Line Fever* to the *Smokey and the Bandit* series, and Chuck Norris's entry, *Breaker! Breaker!,* which teased "He's got a CB radio and a hundred friends who just might get mad!"

CB radio waves connected strangers with a shared destiny and turned them into friends, rolling across America. The CB was a tool that could communicate news in real time about bad weather, ice on the roads, crashes, traffic, and road closures so that others could avoid delays and accidents. It kept truck drivers alert and engaged during long hours on the highway. It tipped them off to the bears and any speed traps, and helped keep America moving.

Convoy members shared meals at America's diners and created their own foodie culture of truck-stop comfort, places where Flo's meat loaf was the food of the gods. The highway diner was the medieval inn of our times, an oasis where travelers met along their journeys, often at the same time every week. Truck drivers drove the economy that kept these places open, and guaranteed that the food was good—there was a lot of competition and a lot of chatter about who had the best cherry pie.

We've seen a loss of the slow ethic of the roads. Chains have moved in where Mom and Pop once made the bacon

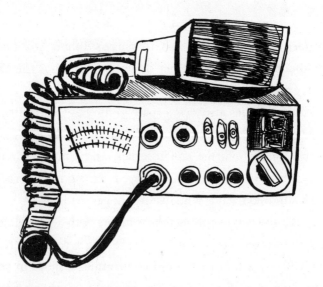

and eggs and pumped the gas. The truck-driving community is changing, and with it, part of a grand American
folklore.

The arrival of the cell phone and new, more technologi-
cally hip modes of communication — and the new laws that
banned any handheld devices for drivers — are helping to
put the kibosh on the CB and its culture. And it's not just
the hip lingo that has disappeared: Think about it, when's
the last time you saw a convoy on the highway?

In the old days it wouldn't be unusual for a trucker to
stop for a troubled motorist — truckers were once known
as the Knights of the Road. Today, with the new time limits
imposed on the industry by the Federal Motor Carrier
Safety Administration, drivers have to drive faster within
fixed time constraints. As of the publication of this book,

the law states that a driver can only drive eleven hours in a fourteen-hour period and then has to take ten hours off. The result is that when they are on the road, they have to drive as fast and as far as they possibly can, and so a rule intended for safety actually has the unintended consequence of forcing drivers to put the pedal to the metal and congregate on the same few fast-moving highways.

I have the fortunate experience of working with Larry Boukal and Cannonball Express, a "less-than-load" carrier based in Omaha. Every pound of what I sell goes on separate pallets in Cannonball Express's red-and-white trucks to cities around the country, every single week. In ten years, the carrier has never made a mistake.

The importance of less-than-load carriers cannot be underestimated—they allow smaller companies to ship anything, even in the smallest increments. While big businesses can fill an eighteen-wheeler with a day's deliveries, smaller businesses like mine need to share truck space. Less-than-load carriers are our saviors.

After hauling ass on America's highways, the national cross-country truckers deliver to local companies— whether it's in New York or Philly or Los Angeles or Santa Fe—where a new set of warriors, including the drivers for FedEx and UPS, do their own dance through the streets.

In Manhattan, the LaFrieda Meats distributor drivers— guys like Checo, Willy, Alex, Danny, and Kevin—drive trucks full of cases of meat over bridges and through tunnels, over crowded, potholed streets jammed with bikers and jaywalkers, cops, and city buses. They maneuver through rain, snow, street fairs, and water-main breaks to get the goods to your favorite downtown restaurants. They weave in and out of traffic like cavaliers, beautiful to watch but largely underappreciated.

So when you see a truck on the highway or on the road, whether it's a Kenworth T800, a FedEx panel truck, or the guys from the Tom Cat bakery delivering the daily bread, show those drivers some love. They have one of the toughest jobs in the world—we'd be at sea without them. Go ahead. Take a look around you. Try to name something in your home, or on your plate, that did not come off a truck.

CHAPTER 24

Carlo Petrini

Action is the foundational key to all success.

—*Pablo Picasso*

Where are the real leaders?

I'm not talking about corporate CEOs, who present annual reports to shareholders, but visionaries, brave warriors, and orators in the mold of Martin Luther King, Jr., John F. Kennedy, Che Guevara, or Winona LaDuke— leaders who can inspire entire movements.

Where is the passion and willingness to stand up for the important issues of our day, without concern for the effect it will have on advertisers, boards of directors, or short-term profits? Where is the leader who fights for the underdog—and actually makes a difference?

It may be true that we don't have battles in front of us that stir the souls of the populace as we did in the civil rights era, or in the fight for women's suffrage, or against the Vietnam War. But the crisis we face now — a planet that is practically suffocating, while our children are practically being force-fed empty calories by corporate conglomerates whose worldview values nothing more than a beefy bottom line — *is* the major issue of our time. A war against fast food may not have the friction that a war against a war does, but if we do not catch that tiger by the tail right now we are facing a future of fewer farms, plastic food, and a national health crisis that promises to explode.

No one has done more to organize and speak out on these issues than Carlo Petrini.

Carlo likes to say that committees destroy all good ideas. Checks and balances and differing opinions help ensure fairness when there is poor leadership, but they can quickly bog things down and hinder grand visions. Carlo is the benevolent monarch of the Slow Food movement, and he uses that power sagely but without compromise to move the organization forward in startling and dynamic ways, launching projects that no one else could ever have imagined.

Even before Slow Food, Carlo had strong leftist beliefs, and his convictions turned him into a political player in his hometown of Bra, in the Piedmont region of Italy. He used the town hall and cafés as his pulpit, waxing poetic, often hilariously, on any political issue or peeve that popped into his head. He was the king of the commedia dell'arte, gesticulating like a mad Italian while he prattled in his Piedmontese dialect, mixing French with mountain Italian, and it had audiences riveted. He changed minds—he was funny, but he always spoke the truth, and the laughter greased the wheels of his message.

He knew, too, that much activism, like the politics it pretended to abhor, had been hampered with bureaucracy and the Chatty Cathys who loved to talk high-minded ideals at the back table of the local bar but too often got nothing done. Carlo, however, was a man of action as much as he was a man of ideas and convictions, and he went into every new challenge headfirst.

Infuriated by the mediocrity and the lack of diversity on the state-run radio, he decided to bust open the airwaves for more music and ideas, and in 1974 he mobilized some equally fired-up friends to launch what would be only the second independent radio station in all of Italy. At the time the Italian government ridiculously claimed that the radio dial could only hold a few stations—effectively prohibiting new stations from starting up and squashing any dissenting voice. Carlo's station, which he christened with the unapologetically communist handle Radio Bra Onde Rosse, used a transmitter he had rescued from an American surplus tank from the Korean War. He broadcast left-wing polemics, talk shows, and the subversive music of the day. He was projustice, feminist, and anticorruption, and strived to be a model of fairness and having fun.

In what now seems like an opera buffa, the Italian government took down the transmitter, only to see Carlo rescue more surplus radio gear and get back on the air blasting

Jefferson Airplane. This happened a few times, until he was finally hauled into court, a grand gesture that backfired when Italian luminaries like actor Roberto Benigni (himself a modern master of the commedia dell'arte) and future Nobel laureate Dario Fo came to testify on Carlo's behalf, making him far more famous than he ever had been and ensuring that his message got out to the largest audience possible.

Carlo's modus operandi was to turn his passions into deeply personal revolutions. One of his great loves was Italian folk music, which was getting short shrift from a society mad with pop, so his next act, after freeing the airwaves, was to launch what would become the largest folk festival in Europe. Modeled after a medieval fertility tradition, in which peasants would walk from farm to farm and perform in return for fresh eggs at the end of winter, Cantè J'euv is a tradition that lives on today.

Carlo was also tuning in to what would be his true calling—he began to realize that the food in Italy was becoming homogenized and lazy. The varieties and quality of bread in the cafés were dwindling. The local cheeses were giving way to a few national favorites. The local viniculture—Barolos, Barberas, and Barbarescos, for instance—were underachieving, while New World wines were being celebrated.

Italy was losing many of its traditions to the rank imperialism of encroaching global brands, and of convenience at any cost. Carlo's energy and drive led him to the presidency of a new regional food organization spun off from ARCI, the Association of Recreation and Creativity in Italy. His new organization was ARCI-GOLA, which more or less translates as "ARCI—throat division." This was the predecessor of Slow Food.

Slow Food started in 1986 with the simple act of Carlo and his buddies eating pasta on the Spanish Steps of Rome, in protest against the first McDonald's in Italy, which opened there. Almost eighty years after the Italian Futurists organized a movement to celebrate the virtues of velocity, machines, and war, Carlo started a countermovement to defend good, clean, and fair food that respected tradition.

He has since grown Slow Food to 100,000 members in 150 countries divided into 1,500 separate chapters. The events his team produces are monumental in scope: The original Salone del Gusto—a veritable amusement park of food—pulled in hundreds of thousands of people to eat and learn, and the Terra Madre event brought five thousand farmers together to talk and network. In the late 1990s Carlo's commitment to ensuring his legacy inspired him to found the University of Gastronomic Sciences, which has educated thousands of students.

Carlo inspired people to fight for the causes that he knew were important to our culture, and he used many of the same tactics that corporations much larger than his band of rebels employed. He understood that it took the same amount of time to get his message out to a thousand people as it did a hundred thousand.

He started a publishing house to produce magazines and books that communicated his mantra of respecting our natural rhythms while promoting quality food, the land, and slow business. Among the most valuable of these was his *Osteria Guide,* which listed descriptions and addresses of mom-and-pop restaurants around Italy that specialize in the local cuisines. And when he arrived at these places, after driving on winding roads for hours to find a small village and some small stone building that housed an old couple who ran the place, he could stir up the same energy as the Rolling Stones once did perpetrating their rock 'n' roll in small clubs and bars.

Carlo coined the term *eco-gastronomy.* He conceived a metaphorical Ark of Taste onto which he boarded foods that were on the brink of extinction. Carlo argued for gastronomy to be treated as a soft science, like anthropology or sociology. He demanded quality and supported the people who could produce it. Education, he argued, was the key.

We can all learn from Carlo, who is bound for a Nobel Prize one day. The sustainable food movement has a bad habit of dragging action down into the tar pits of talking, but he has always shot first and worried later, and has never allowed himself to be stymied by the obstacles tossed at him by naysayers or academics. He knows that slow is great when it comes to food, but that's not how you change the world.

CHAPTER 25

Sex Sells, or, For Every Season There Is a Meat

Live in each season as it passes; breathe the air,
drink the drink, taste the fruit, and resign yourself
to the influence of the earth.

— *Henry David Thoreau*

An industrial farm is a joyless place. Even the studly breeders don't get to have sex! Everything is artificially coerced, and then artificially inseminated. These farms are not idyllic, impressionist paintings of greenery and sunshine — more like the technological nightmare of tubes and machines and vaultlike freezers, racks of test tubes, genetic manipulators, and the cold-hearted tools of a science on the brink of disaster.

Did you ever read Charles Dickens and wonder why they were always eating ducks and geese at Christmastime?

Well, it's because of the sex lives of these toothsome birds. It's that simple. Remember the song "Makin' Whoopee"? *Another season, another reason, for makin' whoopee.* You certainly didn't think that applied only to people, did you?

Just as tomatoes and strawberries are best in the summer, so too do our animal chums have their own seasons, and being tuned in helps teach us respect for the natural order of things—the miracle of Earth orbiting the Sun and giving us the joys of spring, summer, winter, and fall. These days it's not so obvious, in the supermarket, anyway, because all meat is available all the time. But when naturally bred animals are ready for slaughter, in season, that is Earth speaking to us.

Eating meat at its naturally most robust, ready-for-market time of year is part of our covenant as responsible, sustainable, thoughtful, spiritually sound human beings, and it's humbling in a way that makes us all feel part of something much bigger than us.

And when the season strikes, buy these animals in bulk and freeze what you don't eat fresh—to embrace livestock by season means more than just laying out a single lavish holiday meal. You can make it your fashionable protein for weeks. Think sandwiches, and then meat for chili or ragù for your pasta. Almost any animal, including lamb and turkey, makes a great burger, and this is very important—when we only eat prime cuts, it leads to waste. Grinding the cheaper cuts is going to help us achieve an America where small farms can survive, because we are helping them sell the entire beast.

Let's start in fall: In October farms all over the world are exploding—this is harvest season, when the spring's efforts are ready for the table and it's time for us to fatten up for the winter. But at Heritage we're most excited about October's bounty of goats—in fact, we call it Goatober.

Goat is consumed in more places on the planet than any other livestock, with wonderful recipes and traditions representing a mosaic of cultures, although in America it suffers from the lack of a good marketing scheme—no "Where's the beef?" or "the other white meat" to push goat to the forefront of a carnivore's cuisine that has always been dependent on cows and pigs.

Goats are like horny newlyweds down on the farm. They do it like crazy in the fall, and they reproduce easily, usually birthing twins in spring. When fall comes, you either eat them, especially the males that do not produce milk, or you'll have to get them sleeping bags to get through the chilly evenings. They've spent their summers munching on green grass and by early fall they are at their peak, before they get too old, tough, and gamey.

In November, don't be a turkey, eat one! Left to their own instincts, turkeys do it in the late winter and early spring and are ready for harvest in twenty-four weeks, which conveniently turns out to be Thanksgiving, when as a species, they want to be eaten. And that is why the tradition exists. But don't leave it there—you could be eating turkey sandwiches and beautiful turkey breasts and drumsticks right through till Christmas, and don't forget the ground turkey for burgers or chili. We've said it before and we'll say it again, ground meat is what keeps America's independent farmers in business.

Today, of course, turkey sandwiches are everywhere all year round, but nature pushed hard to put that bird on the Pilgrims' table. If you are eating a fresh turkey in July, well, you can bet that turkey was not the product of a satisfying sexual experience—there wasn't a tom anywhere near a female when that bird was conceived.

December is Dickensian and, once again, the time for ducks and geese. For Americans, they may seem a bit Old World and intimidating to cook, but the truth is they are no more difficult to prepare than a chicken or a turkey, and they are an incredibly tasty alternative. Stephen Barber, the chef at Farmstead restaurant in Napa, calls geese "rib eye in the sky" because they are that meaty and wonderful.

January and February are great times to enjoy cured meats, salumi, prosciutto, anything that has been salted and preserved. Why? Because as humans became civilized, this is what we created to survive the winter. Winter is tough— it's why squirrels hoarding nuts set such an apt example for the rest of us. It's why bears hibernate. Winter is about survival. And if the winter lasts into March, you can still gnaw on that prosciutto.

Come spring, when March roars in like a lion, you should be tucking into some lamb. There is a reason that lamb is central to Passover and Easter—or did you think it was just convenient symbolism? Nope, that's when young lambs are ready for the slaughter, based on their natural mating patterns. And it's a good time to eat the older, more mature sheep, too, since they are done breeding or milking and are ready for harvest.

Again, buy in bulk: Many of the country's best lamb and goat farms are not at the level yet where they can break up those animals into pieces and still keep their business viable. Buying a twenty-pound half lamb or goat, butchered to your specs, is the only way to eat the elite at this point in time, and the best way to help the farmer.

Even though cows do it all year long, some cuts are best known during certain seasons: Just look at how many Jewish grandmothers have ruined perfectly good briskets at Passover, overcooking them with ketchup and chemically based dry soup mix. We can't explain why anyone would want to cook like that, but the reason brisket is popular in early spring is that it is a good, lean rough cut, the cut of the cow that stands up and lasts best through the winter until it is the last part of the cow left. It's also no coincidence that we eat corned beef on St. Patrick's Day.

Coming into summer, you'd be a fool not to eat salmon during the wild salmon harvesting season — those are the months you'll get it fresh from Alaska, and you should only ever eat salmon from Alaska (even frozen the rest of the year!), which is the largest wild salmon run in the world. Better not to eat salmon at all than eat their flabby, sad-sack, farm-raised industrial cousins.

More importantly, summer is grilling season. Pigs,

chickens, and cows are incorrigible, they do it all the time. Like rabbits. So sure, you can eat them all year round, but you should try to leave them alone when other animals want eating during the rest of the year. That's a good way to help promote sustainability.

And that is today's lesson: When an animal has its moment, eat it, eat it often, and learn to prepare it in many ways. Celebrate nature, and the traditions we have created around these animals over thousands of years of farming and breeding. Do it because it is healthy and responsible, because it is the natural thing to do, because it is sustainable and succulent.

Cole Porter said it best in "Let's Do It" — *Birds do it, bees do it... They say that roosters do it... With a doodle and cock...* And there you have it. Let our animals be happy. Please, eat them in season. Let them have sex.

CHAPTER 26

Let It Rot

A corpse is meat gone bad. Well and what's cheese?
Corpse of milk.

—*James Joyce*

In America we are obsessed with the new. We bow down
at the altar of youth. We are blinded by shiny objects. We
throw away things that the rest of the world would cherish.

But my family roots are Brazilian—and we have a
good sense of the old, the worn, the lived-in, and especially
what you might call the rotten, because as all Brazilians
know, a banana getting black and smelly in your kitchen's
fruit bowl is the sweetest thing that can happen to breakfast or dessert.

Food tastes best when its essence is concentrated. Imagine a day when food lived in larders and root cellars and not
double-wide stainless steel Fridge-o-Plexes with atomic ice
machines and more compartments than a magician's frock.

Just think about the flavors—the wonderful *putrescence*—that were part and parcel of good eating back then, and that had the added benefit of keeping a community of essential microbes healthy in your gut.

There is a reason why those who can afford to, obsess over when to open a bottle of wine. Like kids who toodle off to college behaving like children and come back four years later demanding to be taken seriously, some bottles need time to find themselves.

There are plenty of foods, like most sane adults, that need a little time left alone—every culture seems to have its favorite form of ultraputrescent delicacy, from Iceland's fetish for smelly shark meat to China's prized hundred-year egg. Kimchi and sauerkraut are best when "cooked" in pots buried underground. And where would New York be without a Lower East Side awash in the stink of pickles?

Even some beers like a little extra time fermenting in the barrel or the bottle. High-sugar beers with heavy flavor profiles—strong Belgian ales, stout, and barley wine—all of them taste deeper and sweeter and take on the flavor of their barrels when given the chance to take a semester off before being poured into a glass.

A good cheesemonger is a merchant of decomposition. Some cheeses can sit in the refrigerator, or just hang out on the counter, for weeks. Every cheese has a perfect age—some cheddars can hold up for up to fifteen years in Wisconsin. Goudas in Holland can be aged for up to eight years. Parmigiano-Reggiano, arguably the world's greatest cheese, is generally aged for two. Only very fresh cheeses like mozzarella are made to be eaten the day they are made.

Along with ancient Bordeaux, dry-aged steak is another obsession of meat lovers with a few bucks to spare, but what is dry aging, really, except letting God have His way with your meat? Ever have a rib eye that's been aged for weeks and weeks and has some funk on it, a mold that stinks like butter and blue cheese?

Even fresh meat should be at room temperature before it is prepared. A little bit of time and the heat of the kitchen help the meat molecules get moving again and open the flavors up like a decanted wine.

There is never a time where there isn't a Surryano ham from Surry, Virginia, produced by my favorite Heritage cure-master, S. Wallace Edwards & Sons, sitting out on my counter. It's the best $200 I spend all year — one ten-pound boneless prosciutto-style ham will create hundreds of memorable snacks.

The beauty of dry-cured ham is that all the moisture has been removed from it during the salting, smoking, and aging process, so it does not need to be refrigerated. You can store it at room temperature for years and eat it whenever. It will never go bad. Maybe after a long time you'll want to slice off the outermost layer, but the mold stops there, and right underneath will be that salty burgundy succulence ready for slicing.

Even your tools should embrace rot. My kitchen prides itself on the crud at the bottom of my Lodge pot. Lodge cookware is made in Tennessee and, according to the hundred-plus-year-old company's instructions, caring for it should involve adding a coat of oil and cooking it right into the pan rather than washing it with soaps and detergents, which seems to contradict everything our modern lives tell us about keeping everything spangled and Scrubbing Bubbles clean.

Why? To keep the iron "seasoned" and protected from moisture. The more you cook, the better it gets. When you maintain and even repair the "seasoning," your cookware can last a century. The goal is to create a gorgeous crust that holds dear the memory of every dish that has come before, and over the years, your pot or skillet will sing, and every piece of meat will come out better for it.

In America we are obsessed with sell-by dates, but so often we are throwing out things that aren't just "still good," they're actually better. We're not advocating drinking milk that has gone off. There is yogurt for that. But good things come with age and time. Trust your food. Let it rot.

CHAPTER 27

Build a Slaughterhouse

Regard it as just as desirable to build a chicken
house as to build a cathedral.

— *Frank Lloyd Wright*

The single biggest obstacle for sustainable and humane
independent animal farms is the lack of USDA-inspected
slaughterhouses and processing facilities. But we've never
understood why opening more facilities is such a problem.

I hear nightmare stories all the time of farmers from
New York to California who have to book eight months in
advance—before they are even sure their livestock will be
ready—just to get on a plant's schedule. And then they have
to drive a day in either direction because there is nothing
closer. To add insult, with the lack of competition, the existing slaughterhouses have little incentive to serve the special
needs of the responsible farmer at a fair price, or to make

good when they make mistakes. Many would-be farmers ultimately don't start farms because of the lack of processing.

But let's face it, building a slaughterhouse isn't all that complex. We build rockets and put pig hearts in human bodies. We do all sorts of ambitious stuff. And yet the lack of slaughterhouses continues to be the number-one topic at every sustainable meat conference.

Our partner slaughterhouse in Missouri, Paradise Locker Meats, started out skinning deer during deer season and grew to be a profitable business every week of the year and a major employer in its town. Anya Fernald opened a successful slaughterhouse in California (designed by Temple Grandin) as part of her Belcampo farm and retail outlets, and is making pasture to plate a tasty reality. This is the kind of infrastructure that should exist outside every major city like a lighthouse for local independent farmers.

It's time to stop kvetching and start chopping. We need knives, not ideas — building a meat-processing plant doesn't cost much more than opening a decent restaurant. And so for everyone who ever gave lip service to the lack of slaughterhouses and processors, here is what you need to get started:

First, you are going to need a few knives. Also something with which to sharpen them. Everyone will need rubber boots, a waterproof apron, serious rubber gloves, a bump cap, a scabbard, and a node hook. This is all personal equipment. Tools of the trade. Easy stuff.

On the kill floor you'll need a few bigger toys: a kill pin, a stunner, some chain hoists, a scalder, a skinning cradle, a scraping table, a gut buggy, hog gambles, a beef spreader, and a couple of no-nonsense saws. A brisket saw and a splitting saw should do. You need a good supply of hot water and lots of hoses. And a sink. A hot rail scale is useful to weigh carcasses, and lots of barrels help haul out the offal.

For processing you are going to need some refrigeration and a rail system—a bit bigger and more complex than a scabbard, but still a far cry from NASA. You need breaking tables, cutting tables, a band saw, a handheld break saw, and some more precise knives to cut pretty steaks. A few other items to put on the Christmas list would be a grinder and stuffer to make ground beef and sausage, a paper wrap dispenser, a Cryovac, and maybe a smokehouse. Hopefully all of this will be available in a future edition of *The Whole Earth Catalog* (see chapter 31).

You'll need some brains and brawn as well—able hands on the floor, and someone who can write an HACCP (Hazard Analysis and Critical Control Points) food safety plan. A high tolerance for blood and guts from all involved wouldn't hurt, either. And some webcams to set an example for the barons of Big Ag who would prefer that their own slaughterhouses not be monitored too closely.

CHAPTER 28

Slow Down

Adopt the pace of nature: her secret is patience.

—*Ralph Waldo Emerson*

The modern condition is one fraught with perilous velocity. Everything, it seems, is moving at the speed of light. We check our phones hundreds of times a day—for e-mail, tweets, and God knows what, as if a sudden bottleneck on the information highway would cripple our ability to navigate our lives.

Once upon a time people gathered in town squares to hear the news. We all knew our neighbors and town leaders. We had steady relationships with our butchers and bakers. We pored over newspapers. It was a "slow" lifestyle, because we had no choice. Time wasn't hypersegmented. We didn't lose our patience if we had to wait more than a few seconds for our Facebook page to load.

The speed of modern life is destroying our ability to see

what is really happening around us. Imagine this: If you were traveling across the countryside by horse and buggy, you would see everything that passed by in great detail. You could admire the high notes of the countryside, and even stop to talk to the people, or smell the flowers. Now imagine you are in a car traveling seventy miles per hour. What do you see? Mostly just a blur. Now imagine you are on a jet plane — you get to where you are going quickly, but without any experience of the journey.

An important part of the food chain is simply easy-going banter at our local shops. Part of the fabric of community is stitched with the time we spend waiting in line with neighbors at the grocery store and making small talk with the guy at the register.

Gastronomic *tétoir* grows slowly. It's based on human contact and the unfettered exchange of ingredients and ideas. Convenience is an agent of destruction! Ordering groceries by phone or Internet may save time, but it is also removing an intimacy that is the backbone of our society. FreshDirect and companies like it, which deliver groceries ordered via Internet, may be easy, but at the cost of our becoming disconnected. Earlier we talked about sleeping with your butcher. This is just fucking him over.

We have become dependent on all the technology that we were told would help us. Our iPhones and mobile devices are like digital prostheses — could we even function if they were taken away, or would we hobble through the day like disabled people, as if suddenly we'd lost a limb?

The less we talk to our neighbors and those within our community, the more isolated we all become, and the closer we come to a complete breakdown of a healthy social structure. Sure, we are all connected through our smartphones, but what are we *really* saying in these short blasts? Is any meaningful communication actually happening? Without human contact, the art of conversation withers on the vine.

CHAPTER 29

Vegetarian, You Have Blood on Your Hands!

Politics is the art of controlling your environment.
—*Hunter S. Thompson*

There are few things we hate more than radicalized vegetarians spewing vitriol against meat eaters as murderers. It's like a crazy person screaming at the rain.

We know that vegetarians have their hearts in the right places, but their argument is a loser. It is truly sad. All that wonderful, fanatical vegetarian energy...wasted! People eat meat like cats eat canaries. Period. And trying to stop that is absurd.

The truth is, if hard-core vegans and vegetarians had put their efforts into fighting for humane farming and not into waging a war against eating animals, or wearing leather, THE CARNIVORE'S MANIFESTO probably would never have been written, and they would have been spared one more salvo against their movement.

Trying to stop evolution is ridiculous. We are carnivores — and have been hunting since we learned to walk on two legs. No amount of singing, dancing, preaching, protesting, or proselytizing is going to stop people from killing and eating animals.

Paul McCartney has written some remarkably optimistic music, but when it comes to his vegetarian politics, Sir Paul has done more harm than good by chirping about a non–meat-eating paradise. He's tilting at windmills. We love the idea of Meatless Mondays, which he promotes, but ultimately he's taken everyone's eyes off the real enemy — the cruelty of corporate farming and the poisoning of our food chain. It's irresponsible, and all it does is help divide and polarize vegetarians and carnivores who could be working together to stop cruelty to animals while supporting an alternative.

And while we're at it, PETA should stop spending money fighting fur — that message has gotten through loud and clear. They are not going to change that many more minds. Their efforts should be geared toward Perdue, Smithfield, Cargill, the oligarchs of Big Ag and cruel factory farming. Those are their enemies. Dumping paint on a socialite in fur doesn't impress me. Embarrass the board of directors at Perdue and I'll write you a check right now.

And enough about foie gras. Seriously, California outlawed foie gras — as if that would have an impact on global eating? What they should have been fighting for is bigger cages for egg chickens, access to sunlight for pigs, and cameras in slaughterhouses, which would have been a big win for everyone.

One example of misguided vegetarian orthodoxy: A restaurant is only considered vegetarian if there is no meat served on the premises at all. The result is "vegetarian restaurants" that serve by-and-large utterly boring, tasteless, mushy hippie gruel. Just because you are "vegetarian" and have some wind flutes on the stereo does not legitimize poorly cooked soba noodles with goopy tahini and a Styrofoam salad.

There is no reason to sacrifice taste and pleasure for a bogus green badge of courage. Any good restaurant should be able to deliver a wonderful, seasonal, delicious, completely vegetarian meal. When vegans come to our radio station at Roberta's Pizza in Brooklyn, we offer them the *pizza rosso*—just tomato sauce and garlic, totally vegan and completely delicious.

One more thing: Quit calling tofu "turkey dogs" or "sausages" or "burgers." It's worse than nonalcoholic beer. It confuses the message to the converted, and the pretense annoys everyone.

We love vegetables—as we've said before, if fast food were all that was available, we'd go down the herbivore path, too. In fact, if you consider how much we rail against factory-farm and commodity meat, THE CARNIVORE'S MANIFESTO is probably the single greatest argument for vegetarianism ever published.

Want to make a serious change toward a more humane food chain? Quit trying to build a moral high ground on top of a pile of quinoa and sprouts—vegetarians and omnivores need to work together for the ethical treatment of animals.

CHAPTER 30

Take Back Lunch

I've never met a woman in my life who would give
up lunch for sex.

— *Erma Bombeck*

The midday meal is like a black hole in the world of slow
and sustainable food. Every day, even the most strident
among us — at least those of us with jobs — are faced with a
steeplechase of fast-faster-fastest options when that lunch
bell rings.

Lunch is the gauntlet that God has thrown down to test
our resolve. Subway! Wendy's! Two-slices-and-a-Coke, five
bucks! It's time to just say no.

Fast food is a national plague. Even in chic neighborhoods, if you haven't brown-bagged it you are faced with
delicious but dubious options: sandwich shops and salad
bars, all peddling victuals of unknown provenance, and of
course the ubiquitous chain restaurants that pockmark

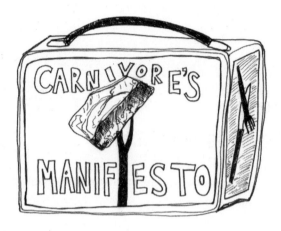

America like acne. Corporate cafeterias might offer a patina of thoughtful quality—Quiche! Short rib! Three-cheese mac and cheese! And a vegetarian option!—but who knows where it all comes from? That low-fat Boar's Head turkey may look more appealing than the goopy Salisbury steak, but that turkey lived a miserable life, you can count on it. It's important to research and read labels and look for the things that are important to you—organic, no preservatives, no additives, pasture-raised.

Twenty years ago our options were slim, but now with the great energy that surrounds the food scene we can all effect a change. The landscape is ripe with greenmarkets and responsible sandwich makers and food trucks peddling organic meals.

When you find a place that can deliver good, clean, and fair food, go out of your way to go there, and go there often, and let those restaurants and vendors who aren't on board know that you'd love to give them your business, too, just as soon as they get with the program. Encourage your coworkers to join the takeover. Storm the gates of your universities and corporate cafeterias and let them know you demand more fresh, local food. And if you are in a place where these niceties aren't so readily available, a lunch box is your ticket to the revolution. Pack it with real cutlery and real napkins, righteous food, dessert, maybe sneak in half a bottle of wine, and I guarantee it will be contagious—watch as your coworkers and colleagues compete with their own cool lunch boxes, from retro *Brady Bunch* and *Dukes of Hazzard* models to sleek brushed-aluminum affairs, but all containing the ticket to taking back lunch.

If we could all commit to eating better lunches even as often as once a week, a myriad of worthy farms and businesses would blossom, and the effects would be felt across generations while unhealthy, nonsustainable options withered for lack of business.

But it's up to us as fellow travelers on the slow train to deliver the gospel.

CHAPTER 31

Remember *The Whole Earth Catalog*!

Where is the wisdom we have lost in knowledge?
Where is the knowledge we have lost in
information?

   —*T. S. Eliot*

Once upon a time, before we all walked around with computers in our pockets, finding information was often clumsy and difficult. There used to be "phone booths," and in these phone booths were giant directories— "phone books"—in which one could look up "phone numbers," assuming all the pages were still intact and that it was the correct directory in the first place.

There were books and guides for all sorts of stuff. It was a time when highway maps were large and difficult to fold, let alone navigate. They were so big and unwieldy that people crashed their cars trying to read them while driving.

People had to go to libraries to do their homework, and if the book you needed wasn't there, you were out of luck. The idea that information was always at your fingertips was science fiction fantasy, the stuff of Asimov or Roddenberry. And the people who collected information were a rare breed. It was a difficult job with no romance. It was a grind.

One of the greatest and without a doubt most progressive directories of all time was *The Whole Earth Catalog*.

"When I was young, there was an amazing publication called *The Whole Earth Catalog*," Steve Jobs once marveled during a commencement speech at Stanford University. "One of the bibles of my generation...It was sort of like Google in paperback form, thirty-five years before Google came along. It was idealistic and overflowing with neat tools and great notions."

It was indeed a thing to behold—quite literally awesome in ways that no longer even exist. The cover featured one of the first photos of the planet Earth taken from space to be made public by NASA, something of a coup during a cold war that fought to keep secret even our peaceful satellite capabilities. The book itself was almost two feet tall, like a monolith left by ancient astronauts, and the typesetting was insane, with more moving parts than a space shuttle.

Flipping through an old edition now sends the mind

reeling: page 285 has an ad for old-fashioned sailing din-ghies sold by the Old Boathouse in Seattle. Page 207 offers a Porta-Shower for $24.95: "A good bus shower, or for scarce-water situations, or where the river's too cold." Just $7.50 got you a book called the *Museum of Early American Tools*. *The Edible Native Plants of the Rocky Mountains* cost $10. You could buy cassettes of old radio shows, marbles, or space blankets that kept you warmer than wool, or a key to read-ing hieroglyphics. There were primitive synthesizers and adding machines—the height of technology!—plus druggy underground comics. You could spend a week just reading the thing.

But it was all about mail order, and bringing people closer to these tools. *The Whole Earth Catalog* opened up new, slow possibilities and options for anyone who could work an envelope and a stamp.

The intro to the first edition, published DIY (slow!) style in 1968, spelled it out:

> We are as gods and might as well get good at it. So far, remotely done power and glory—as via government, big business, formal education, church—has succeeded to the point where gross defects obscure actual gains. In response to this dilemma and to these gains a realm of intimate, personal power is developing—power of the indi-vidual to conduct his own education, find his own inspiration, shape his own environment, and share

his adventure with whoever is interested. Tools that aid this process are sought and promoted by the WHOLE EARTH CATALOG.

The Whole Earth Catalog was a self-proclaimed "evaluation and access device. With it, the user should know better what is worth getting and where and how to do the getting."

This wasn't the Yellow Pages—you couldn't buy your way in. This was not eBay, or a Top 100 list, and it wasn't built on anonymous comments. Each *WEC* listing included a signed recommendation—like a seal of approval, and if the product or vendor didn't maintain its high standards, it was out. *WEC* was not just an aggregator, but an arbiter. That it was community reviewed and that every item was approved by a Whole Earth editorial board put it beyond reproach.

Given all our technology today, we are amazed that we have nothing even close to this guide—a peer-reviewed clearinghouse of tools for progressive and alternate lifestyles, an aggregate of the best of the best with a kind and slow focus, compiled by a respected editor and updated frequently. It would be immune to click trends and unqualified reviews, fake Yelpers, planted Amazon reviews, and the false outrage and one-upmanship of bored bloggers.

A new *Whole Earth Catalog*—whether print or online—needs to offer its readers the tools to foment revolution. The food revolution, especially, needs this now—one-stop shopping for the highest-quality sausage stuffers, meat grinders, canning jars, mortars and pestles, fermenting pots, seeds, and breeding stock. Skinning cradles, immersion circulators, esoteric distilling and brewing gear, guides to bathtub chemistry, centrifuges, rotary evaporators, and liquid nitrogen dewars. All of which would make for some mighty good bathroom browsing, but the aim, as with the original *WEC*, would be to help make the reader less dependent on corporate vendors and more self-empowered, actualized, and sustainable. And better yet, these tools would be available direct from the source without having to give a third-party vendor an unearned cut.

On the back cover of the "farewell edition" of *WEC* in 1971 there was a message, which Steve Jobs quoted in his Stanford speech. It said, "Stay foolish, stay hungry."

CHAPTER 32

Consider the Turkey

We can judge the heart of a man by his treatment of animals.

—*Immanuel Kant*

Like Columbus Day—brought to you by the same people who brought you the Spanish Inquisition and were responsible for the expulsion of the Jews from Spain—Thanksgiving is a holiday when it is just more convenient to forget about the sins of the Puritans who came to our shore. Better to let the unfettered light of American providence shine on thee.

But first, consider the turkey. Take a look at the bird that may soon be on your plate.

Turkeys are *the* American bird. Ben Franklin famously mused why the turkey and not the bald eagle should be the symbol of our nation: "For the Truth the Turkey is in Comparison a much more respectable Bird, and withal a true original Native of America," he wrote. "He is besides, though a little vain & silly, a Bird of Courage, and would not hesitate to attack a Grenadier of the British Guards who should presume to invade his Farm Yard with a red Coat on."

Back when the Pilgrims were getting ready for the first Thanksgiving, turkeys ran wild and had to be caught with a trap or by some other clever shenanigan. But the bird most Americans know, the one they are going to cook for T-Day, was hatched in a giant space-age incubator on a huge industrial farm. And its life went downhill from there.

A few days after hatching—in the first of many unnatural and painful indignities—the industrially raised bird has its upper beak and toenails cut off in what can be described charitably as nonelective surgery.

A turkey is normally a very discriminating eater. Left to its own devices, it will search out the exact food it likes and wants to eat, which generally includes insects, grass, and seeds. Turkeys love acorns and nuts. But unfortunately, none of that is on the menu.

Clipping the beak transforms that bird's face into a kind of disfigured shovel—and with a suck hole where a sharp, tool-like beak used to be, all the bird can do is gorge on the superfattening corn-based mash that it is offered. Given their druthers, turkeys would never eat such crap.

And their toenails? They're removed so that the birds can't get into a fracas with the other turkeys, with which they are crowded in the concentration camp–like conditions that are the status quo of modern factory farming.

After their beaks and claws are clipped, mass-produced

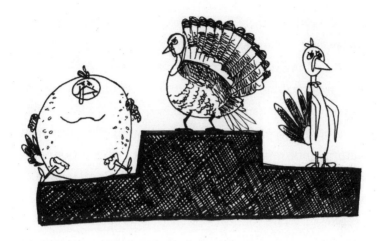

turkeys spend the first three weeks of their lives confined with hundreds of other birds in what is known as a brooder, a heated room where they are kept warm and dry while they grow into adult birds.

The next rite of passage comes in the fourth week, when turkeys reach puberty and grow feathers. For centuries, it was at this point that a humanely raised farm turkey would move outdoors for the rest of its life. But with the arrival of factory turkey farming in the 1960s, any chance of a commodity turkey getting some fresh air went right out the window.

Factory-farm turkeys never see the outdoors. Instead, as many as ten thousand turkeys—all hatched at the same time—are herded from the brooders into a giant, fully automated "grow-out" barn. These barns are generally windowless and are illuminated by bright lights twenty-four hours a day, to mess with the turkeys' heads and keep them awake and eating.

Not only do these birds have no room to move around in the barn, they have no way to indulge their primal instincts, like roosting. Instead, the turkeys are forced to rest in unhealthy, unnatural positions—kind of like sleeping sitting up or standing for you or me.

And they spend their miserable lives in the barn not on natural grass or anything resembling it but on wood shavings, laid down to absorb the overwhelming amount of waste that the flock produces. The ammonia fumes alone would incinerate your eyes. Even at those operations where the top level of the wood shavings is scraped away during the flock's time in the barn, the air is unfit to breathe by any living thing.

Industrial turkeys pay a high price to fulfill the desire of consumers for lots of white breast meat. By their eighth week, these turkeys are severely overweight. Their breasts become so large that they are unable to walk. They cannot breed without assistance, which of course is an indication that every one of them was the product of artificial insemination.

The roughly 270 million turkeys raised in these conditions on factory farms each year are all the same variety, the aptly named Broad Breasted White, which has been developed for a single trait at the expense of all others: producing disproportionately large amounts of white meat in as little time as possible.

Every bit of natural instinct and intelligence has been bred out of these turkeys, so much so that they are famously stupid—to the point where farmers joke that they'll drown themselves by looking up at the rain.

No Broad Breasted White could hope to survive in nature. These turkeys' immune systems are weak from the start from being pushed to grow too fast, and to prevent even the mildest pathogen or disease from killing them, farmers add servings of subtherapeutic antibiotics to their feed. But it is hardly enough to stave off the respiratory problems, heart disease, and joint pains that result from being raised in such brutal conditions without exercise or proper nutrition. The health of these turkeys is so delicate that the few humans who come in contact with them have to wear masks for fear of infecting *the turkeys*.

On nonindustrial farms, it takes turkeys twenty-four weeks to arrive at slaughter weight—about fifteen pounds for a hen and twenty-four pounds for a tom. Industrial turkeys, however, need half that time. By twelve to fourteen weeks, the whole flock is ready for the slaughterhouse.

And while they may boast more meat than a chemical-free heritage breed raised in humane conditions, they are so flavorless as to make this method of breeding little more than an experiment in cruelty.

And so, once slaughtered, the turkeys have to suffer one more indignity before arriving in your grocer's meat case. Because of the monstrous confluence of eating a gruel-like diet designed only to put weight on the birds, and growing up in an environment void of any of the usual things that God likes to contribute to the healthy raising of animals, e.g., fresh air and sunlight, their flesh is so bland and often so mealy that processors need to inject them with saline solution and vegetable oils, improving "mouthfeel" while at the same time artificially increasing shelf life and goosing their weight so they can sell the birds for a few bucks more.

If you are cooking one of these birds for your family, you have to go to heroic lengths to try to counteract the turkey's crackerlike dryness and lack of flavor. Cooks must brine, marinate, deep-fry, and hide the taste with maple syrup, barbecue sauce, and an insane catholicon of herbs, spices, butter, and olive oil. It's no surprise that side dishes have moved to the center of the Thanksgiving menu!

Even so, 45 million turkeys will be sold this Thanksgiving, so turkey producers aren't doing badly for themselves. But the rise of the Broad Breasted White means that dozens of other turkey varieties, including the Bourbon Red, Narragansett, and Jersey Buff, have been pushed to the brink of extinction. With so much cheap commodity turkey filling the supermarket aisles and being promoted so aggressively, there is hardly a market left for heritage breeds and no incentive for farmers to grow them, a great problem for our national gastronomy and for the biodiversity needed for a safe food supply. So if your turkey lists its home address as Butterball, Jennie-O, Cargill, Perdue, Farbest Foods, Prestage Farms, House of Raeford, Foster Farms, West Liberty, Sara Lee, or any of America's industrial bird factories, think twice—and as you shop, you need to look beyond labels like "organic" and "naturally raised." Those are buzz-words that have been co-opted by big business and are no guarantee of a healthier and more humanely raised bird. It's not always easy to get to the bottom of it all, but the question to ask is, Was that turkey raised humanely?

If the person behind the counter where you buy your turkey can tell you about the farm and the farmer who raised it, you are taking a step in the right direction. And you will wind up with a turkey that tastes, well, like a turkey.

CHAPTER 33

We Answer to a Higher Authority

To live outside the law, you must be honest.
— *Bob Dylan*

Bob Dylan sang those words in his song "Absolutely Sweet Marie" on his *Blonde on Blonde* album, though he probably boosted the riff from the great Don Siegel noir *The Lineup:* "When you live outside the law, you have to eliminate dishonesty."

Heritage Foods works with sixty independent farmers with no written contracts. We do $10 million of business a year on handshake agreements, and it works because we are all honest. Lawyers will tell you that you need them to function, but when it comes to the food world — or any grassroots, artisanal crafts movement — it's about face-to-face, person-to-person. Integrity is the rule of law in this universe. Suing an Amish farmer is a fool's errand, anyway.

When Mark Ladner placed the first wholesale order

with Heritage in 2005, he was coloring outside the lines—
our contract was nothing more than a firm handshake and
a warning not to fuck it up. And if we didn't, he'd be there
to buy lots of pork and help support our network of farmers, who were growing animals based on his initial commitment. We didn't—fuck it up, that is—and he and his
coconspirators Mario Batali and Joe Bastianich became
anchor customers.

Back then we didn't have the infrastructure that we
needed to fulfill a handful of orders, let alone run a business
as ambitious as ours was. We were young and idealistic
and, frankly, naïve. But our Slow Food colleague Jim
Weaver had a restaurant in New Jersey and let us get a pallet of meat delivered to him every Monday night, and every
Tuesday we were there with a U-Haul to pick up and deliver
the goods.

Delivering fresh pork in the middle of summer in an
unrefrigerated panel truck violated every food safety plan
ever written, but it wasn't like our food sat in the heat. We
had lots of ice and we drove like maniacs. We weren't cutting corners; in fact, our goal was to push the quality envelope while helping independent farmers. But we had to
fly under the radar in the early days to get it done. We broke
a few rules, and everyone from farmer to chef was complicit
in our conspiracy.

I saw this rule-breaking ethos prosper with the nascent
Slow Food, and I saw it when our friends built Roberta's out
of an old auto body shop and insisted they were the future.

The organic revolution began in Alice Waters's kitchen, against all odds and in the most unlikely place. These revolutionaries lived on the fringe with the faith that they were fighting the good fight. And this is how the sustainable food movement exists—through intense honesty and loyalty among a group of would-be outlaws, people who do whatever it takes to see a good mission succeed.

Anybody and everybody who ever stiffed us was excommunicated from the group, and the word got out that they were poison—because none of us can afford to let anyone else get burned. For this movement to move forward, to progress, we have to hold ourselves to standards that are cosmically ahead of the capitalist curve.

CHAPTER 34

I Am a Goat

It's not bragging if you can back it up.
—*Muhammad Ali*

When you are as great as I am, it's hard to be humble.

How is it that I am not the most common livestock found in America? Why do you treat me like a bastard stepchild? Why are you always taking cows and chickens to the dance? MEEEEEHHE!!!!

While you've been whining about corn-eating cattle and oil-dependent, pesticide-rich corporate farmers fucking up the environment, I've been healthy and happy as a clam eating whatever is lying around: stems, twigs, brush, leaves, weeds, grass, shrubs, even poison ivy. And I can climb anywhere, even the sides of mountains, to get to it. Try getting some fat-ass cow to do that.

I fight forest fires by eating undergrowth. I can stand

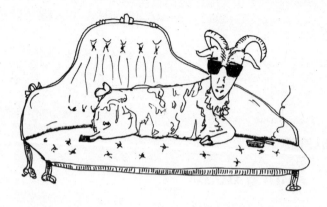

on my hind legs to get to almost anything. George Orwell saw it and wrote a book about it.

I am the answer to all your agriculture problems. I produce half a gallon of milk a day. Worldwide, more people drink my milk than cow's milk. And the cheese? Humboldt Fog, Kunik, Lake's Edge, and Goat Tomme. Baby, I can't lose with the stuff I use!

I am the animal behind Fifth Avenue cashmere, which grows under my chinny-chin-chin. Did you ever wonder where that mohair sweater comes from, that mod bit of couture that that keeps you warm and looking sharp in winter?

I am your farm's MVP. I'm famous for helping other animals. I can break out of a barn during a fire because I paid attention during the safety presentation and remember where the exits are. The rest of the animals rely on me to save their sorry butts.

I'm svelte, not fat, a perfect size six. I'm so pretty even

my poop is fantastic—little round unmuddy turds that are the envy of the animal kingdom.

My breeds are famous, noble, honorable, and celebrated: Arapawa, San Clemente, Tennessee Fainting, Nigerian Dwarf, Oberhasli, LaMancha, Nubian, Toggenburg, Saanen, Pygmy, Kiko, Scandinavian Ridgeback Mountain, and Boer.

I am adaptable and smart. I can live pretty much anywhere, even in a backyard in Brooklyn. I make an awesome pet, although I'm gonna need another goat around. We're social like that.

I am the most fertile, virile, and prolific animal you have ever seen—goats are prone to birthing twins or triplets. And the moment I am born, I'm ready for action—no lying around for years trying to figure shit out like humans.

Pigs are ridiculous! I read that "I Am a Pig" piece and it made me gag. Sure, everyone loves bacon, but faux humility and navel-gazing make me sick.

And birds? You gotta be fucking kidding me. You think Daffy and Donald are the funniest livestock? Think again, dumbass. I'm the funny one. When your girlfriend has a beard, you sort of have to be.

CHAPTER 35

Share the Shit

The ambition for broad acres leads to poor farming, even with men of energy. I scarcely ever knew
a mammoth farm to sustain itself; much less to
return a profit upon the outlay. I have more than
once known a man to spend a respectable fortune
upon one; fail and leave it; and then some man of
more modest aims, get a small fraction of the
ground, and make a good living upon it. Mammoth farms are like tools or weapons, which are
too heavy to be handled. Ere long they are thrown
aside, at a great loss.

—*Abraham Lincoln*

Hopefully we are all past throwing soda cans out the win-
dows of our cars, or leaving cigarette butts on the beach,
but a little reminder to help keep the planet clean is always
in order.

Long after the environmentalist cartoon owl and the crying highway-side Native American have left the building, all of us, except perhaps the most cookie-headed imbeciles and look-the-other-way conservatives, should recognize that we are spoiling our nest. The Industrial Revolution brought us marvels and efficiencies that transformed our lives, but the price has too often been scorched earth and no remorse—pesticide residues are poisoning our rivers and the Gulf of Mexico, rain forests are being destroyed in South America. And corporate farming has left in its wake a brown skid mark the size of California.

A factory farm is like a small city with thousands of pooping citizens. But unlike the civilized model, the common factory farm isn't held to any safe or sensible standard when it comes to processing its waste. These farms pour animal waste into giant man-made lagoons, literally swamps made of hot, wet shit.

There is so much manure that the fields of eastern North Carolina, for instance—where ten million hogs are being bred for slaughter at any given time—cannot absorb all the waste, and it is poisoning the groundwater and contaminating drinking wells. Waste lagoons, some as big as eight acres across, have burst, sending out tsunamis of pig shit, saturating fields, poisoning rivers, and killing thousands upon thousands of fish and other wildlife. And humans are getting sick, too.

Can you imagine if I came over to your house and took a dump in your living room, and turned the place where you play Xbox with your kids into a biohazard hot zone? It's kind of the same thing, the very definition of insanity.

The obvious way to lessen the deadly environmental impact is, to coin a phrase, to share the shit. More farms are essential—ten million hogs is too many for the North Carolina ecosystem, even if the corporate masters were responsibly processing the waste. Which they are not.

So think about this when you are buying meat from the Industrial Food Complex. It's not just bad for you, it's bad for the planet. They are crapping in our homes, and someone is going to have to clean it up. And until they start mailing toxic hog turds along with their dividends, arguing in terms of shareholder value is not an acceptable excuse.

CHAPTER 36

Healthy Animals Don't Need Medicine

Health is the state about which medicine has nothing to say.

— *W. H. Auden*

Seventy percent of the world's antibiotics are being pumped into factory-farmed animals.

That doesn't scare you?

It's very simple: Antibiotics are a sign of sick and weakened, immunodeficient livestock, and eating and even handling these animals put our health in danger, too.

Our question to the Industrial Food Complex is, Are you really such lousy farmers, are you so completely incapable of raising healthy animals, that you have to jack them with chemicals the second they are born? How on earth did this become acceptable?

Factory-farmed animals today come from dangerously manipulated genetics that create breeds that grow much faster than nature intended. The effect is musculoskeletal problems, metabolic disease, and cardiovascular problems — while the animal is getting obese, its systems can't catch up and it needs medicine to keep it alive.

Meanwhile, the results of humans' interaction with antibiotic-ridden meat are mutations that lead to medicine losing its efficacy. This interaction is also killing the diversity of the approximately 100 trillion bacteria that live deep in the coils of our intestines, bacteria that, as Michael Pollan explains, exert a profound influence on our health — almost as great as the genes we inherit from our parents. These bacteria can help humans keep obesity and chronic disease at bay, as well as some infections and food-related illness.

We see a lot of labels like "natural" — which means next to nothing — and "no hormones" on factory-farmed chicken, which is bunk, because it is illegal to use hormones in chickens (cattle, sadly, are another story). But what we want to see is the unambiguous promise of No Antibiotics!

Americans must demand meat that has not been fed antibiotics as part of the routine. Given the economy of scale of commodity farming, we would hope the price increase would be minimal. But if it costs more, we're happy to eat less, but better, safer, tastier, healthier meat.

It is very simple — we do not want medicine in our meat. It is absurd, and dangerous. Corporations have to become better farmers.

CHAPTER 37

National Farmers' Day

I believe a leaf of grass is no less than the journey-work of the stars.

—*Walt Whitman*

We demand that the president of the United States, with the full support of the United States Congress, declare a National Farmers' Day to celebrate the people responsible for our agriculture—past, present, and future.

There are only eleven federal holidays—Thanksgiving, Martin Luther King, Jr.'s birthday, Presidents' Day, Memorial Day, Independence Day, and Veterans' Day among them. But we need one more, to celebrate and remember the people who feed us. Even that out-of-shape groundhog popping out of its hole and predicting the weather gets more play than our farmers.

We propose that Farmers' Day should occur on August 1, the beginning of the slowest-in-spirit month of the year.

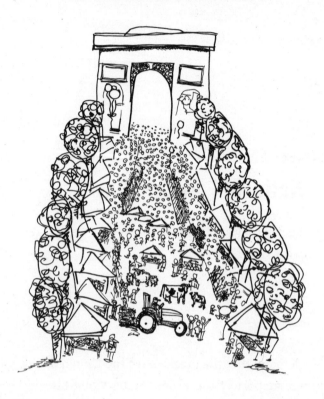

It will be a day for farmers to come to the city and for city dwellers to travel to the farm, all in an effort to connect Americans with the heroes behind our food supply.

Everyone is welcome, from the people of Kansas City and the Carolinas, Texas and Memphis, who party low and slow, to San Francisco vegans, Brooklyn foodies, and all manner of omnivores—all of us will band together to celebrate the American farmer and Earth's bounty!

Every culture we can think of has a harvest day except America, and no, Thanksgiving, our national day of quasi-religious thanks, does not count. We have become too disconnected from the seasons, from a sense of place, from a time when foods were not available all year round.

National Farmers' Day will be a chance to taste new food and get closer to the earth. Most importantly, it is for children, who should learn where their food comes from and should enjoy a curiosity about and respect for what they eat.

We see livestock competitions and farm dinners across the country! Trendy butter churners, urban farmers, chic butchers, and vanguard bakers, basking in the glory of American tradition! This is a time to promote a new wave of agritourism, celebrating Amish farms and amber waves of grain, orchards, ranches, and vineyards. And there shall be a federal mandate for the sun to shine!

National Farmers' Day is a day for hayrides, horseback rides, and kids' rides in goat carts. Egg tossing, potato sack races, bobbing for apples, milking and petting animals, barn raisings, and pie-eating contests. On Farmers' Day animals will parade down Fifth Avenue and cities will blossom into greenmarkets. It will be a time for feasting, and for farmers to be honored at the restaurants where they sell their food.

But to rebuild our food culture and guarantee that our children will grow up embracing healthy, natural food, we'll have to be vigilant to keep the Industrial Food Complex from co-opting the event as publicity for corporate agriculture—know that they will come in sheep's clothing, but inwardly they are as ravening wolves.

We are a nation raised on the backs of our farmers, and National Farmers' Day will celebrate the traditions of our very best foods while promoting a healthy future secured by American independent farmers, the hardest-working people in the world.

CHAPTER 38

Put Your Money Where Your Mouth Is

The world is moved along, not only by great
shoves of its heroes, but also by the aggregate of
the tiny pushes of each honest worker.

—*Helen Keller*

It always strikes me as kind of twisted that when people
think of investing money they think of Charles Schwab, or
some interest-bearing widget being peddled by a corporate
bank whose current track record is plainly atrocious. And
not only because it backed a quintillion bad loans and is complicit in all but tanking the economy of the United States, but
also because it can't even cop to a dollop of culpability. Banks
and investment firms are the poster children for greed.

The entire financial industry has at least trace elements
of Bernie Madoff in its bloodstream. The whole racket has a

whiff of corruption, and it's no wonder—they want to win at the expense of all else and will do anything to turn a profit, to show an increase on the quarterly report and see it reflected in their whackadoo end-of-year bonus, which has so little to do with reality you'd think they were in the LSD business.

In the old days, corporate America represented security and strength. These days, even mighty financial firms teeter at the brink of the abyss. The people we've been told to trust with our money don't actually do or deal in anything real, just profit reports. And we are paying for their financial jiggery-pokery—they can artificially inflate a company's value or make you take a hit for the benefit of other accounts within their own firm. Ultimately, you don't really matter to them.

Why should it give you any sense of confidence to invest with people you have never met and companies you don't know? And even if your fund manager or broker is a pal, and even if you are getting a decent return, you might find that you are investing in companies whose politics disgust you.

So what is the alternative? Stay local. Invest in your community. We've said it before and we'll say it again: Slow food is slow business. The guy down the street whose restaurant is kicking ass and who's looking for a cash injection to expand—that's the guy you want to invest in. And then go and have dinner in your investment and feel great.

Community-supported agriculture (CSA) is by far the

most accessible and practical way for Americans to participate. CSA means basically buying a share of a local farmer's
produce before the season starts, and every week your divi-
dend comes in the form of fresh food. Your destinies are
now wonderfully intertwined.

Slow food is people. Not the same way that *Soylent
Green* is people ("soylent green" being what the government feeds the masses in the 1973 Charlton Heston sci-fi
flick, in which meals made from recalcitrant humans are
used to quell food riots), but an integral part of the schema
nonetheless.

We are only as strong as our farmers, merchants, purveyors, restaurants, markets, and other businesses that sell
and promote the ethical, sustainable, and humanely delicious. Right now we're writing this at Calexico in Brooklyn, which is about to open up two new locations, and we're
wondering how we can get in on the ground floor.

To help us start Heritage Foods, four men looking to
invest some dough gave us $60,000 each. Why? They could
have thrown it into the stock market or a bond or some
fancy fund, but they chose us because they wanted to be
part of a community profit center and take responsibility
for something ethical and positive. Also, they really like
pork chops, and you cannot beat the perks of being a principal in a meat purveyor—that's food for life. Try putting a
number on that. Beats 2 percent interest, that's for sure.

CHAPTER 39

Revolutionaries Wanted, Inquire Within

To every action there is always an equal and opposite reaction.

—Newton's Third Law of Motion

Who will be the next Upton Sinclair or Eric Schlosser? Who will be the freedom fighter who goes behind the castle walls and comes back with a turn on *The Jungle* or *Fast Food Nation*, a missive so incendiary and damning that it will bring corporate farming to its knees as Americans turn their backs on cruelty and chemicals and demand safe, healthy food?

This movement needs revolutionaries of all stripes, from earnest muckrakers to outraged anarchist students staging sit-ins in their cafeterias, demanding fair, clean, humanely farmed food. We need the old-fashioned Yippie

pie-throwers who reward evil politicians with a faceful of meringue. We need monkey-wrenchers to block trucks delivering pain in the form of industrially farmed chickens and to chain themselves to the fences of factories that push pig feces into our rivers.

We need journalists, op-ed writers, and Jane Jacobses who will haunt town council meetings and push back against the cultural imperialism of chain stores and restaurants that eat at our neighborhoods and squeeze out our local businesses. Laws against the incursion of chains have already been passed in tony Nantucket, San Francisco, and Utah, to name but three locales where the citizens have banded together with righteous indignation on their side.

We must vote for politicians who are not weaklings when it comes to the environment, pushovers for big business when it comes to keeping our air and water clean, climate-change deniers destined for the scrap heap of history. Anyone who knowingly dumps poison into a river should go to jail. Period. Stockholders must press against the CEOs and boards of directors—if you own even one share, you have a voice.

We need parents and teachers to take control of our children's futures and push back against the predatory marketing practices of McDonald's, soda companies, cereal makers, and other peddlers of habit-forming empty calories. Our children need to be taught that Ronald is an evil clown!

We all must be united—everyone is self-actualized, capable, and connected through social media. Anyone can educate, infiltrate, and subvert the status quo.

We've said it before: There is no way that Americans at large are ever going to achieve a 100 percent organic lifestyle, but we must all do our part to move the dial away from a cruel factory-farming system and fatty, salty, and sweet processed junk.

Ultimately, there is no better place to fight back against the evils of the Industrial Food Complex than at your own table, with your own family. Let your kitchen be our Lexington and your pantry be our Concord! The revolution begins at home, and that's why, even if you can't raise an army of activists, we challenge you to change just one mind. Perhaps you can convince your rich brother-in-law that feeding his kids processed food every day is a bad idea. THE CARNIVORE'S MANIFESTO is not about assuaging a liberal guilty conscience; it is about eating better, feeling better, and having more fun—remind him that good, fresh food is not only the road to a healthier future for his kids, but it also goes better with his fine wine than the supermarket crap he is in the habit of eating. This is the ultimate, superfocused, and most effective way to practice the old mantra "Think globally, act locally."

CHAPTER 40

Ted Turner

I have a fantasy where Ted Turner is elected president but refuses because he doesn't want to give up power.

—Arthur C. Clarke

Leaders of the sustainable food movement are too often misguided about what real success is. I love hearing stories of Manhattan caterers who buy a whole cow for an event, but if we are ever going to make a genuine difference in the way we eat and the way we show respect for our planet, we need to think bigger, on an enormous, not-so-precious scale that can go mano a mano with the dark side of the Industrial Food Complex.

Ted Turner is best known as a media mogul, the mind behind CNN and the concept of the cable television "superstation." The superstation challenged the monopoly of the Big Three networks—subverting the long-established status quo of the television landscape—and he used this opportunity to broadcast environmental documentaries along with the sports and syndicated sitcoms. His celebrity as a self-made billionaire looms large, as does his infamy for controversial sound bites and his failed bid to take over professional wrestling. But as an environmentalist, he has few peers.

Turner was close friends with Jacques Cousteau and invested millions to keep Cousteau's *Calypso* crew sailing in the Amazon and around the world so that they could continue their important research. The footage of Cousteau aired on Turner's television stations. In addition, Turner's Cartoon Network created programs for children like *Captain Planet and the Planeteers,* which painted polluters and ecological villains in the same colors as Darth Vader and Dr. No.

As a businessman first, Ted Turner teaches us that something is sustainable only if it is actually sustainable—meaning it doesn't lose money. Anything else is just a hobby. And he has been successful as an eco-investor on a planetary level by spectacularly reintroducing native bison to the American West, a phenomenal accomplishment for our collective heritage.

Thanks to Turner's success in the business world, he was able to purchase fifteen ranches across seven states covering almost two million acres, while implementing conservation easements to ensure that they remain open and protected.

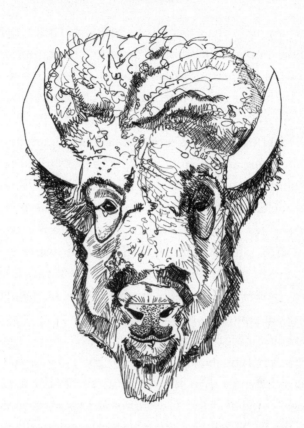

The 170 square miles of Montana's Flying D Ranch are home base for Turner and many of his fifty-six thousand head of bison, a herd that makes him the undisputed poobah of the beast. Roughly one in nine bison in this country live on Turner lands.

Turner has managed to vertically integrate his bison program by finding a trustworthy abattoir in Colorado and opening a restaurant chain called Ted's Montana Grill, where you can get bison nachos, burgers, and steaks. Today there are more than forty Ted's Montana Grills, and by 2021 the number will double. Thanks to Turner, Americans are eating 100 percent grass-fed bison and saving the animals in the process, an essential irony of THE CARNIVORE'S MANIFESTO.

Turner has made his properties a breeding ground for healthy bison, and also for other species that thrived before the white man arrived and began shooting everything in sight, including grizzlies, wolves, mountain lions, bobcats, lynx, coyotes, foxes, bighorn sheep, wolverines, elk, moose, mule deer, whitetails, pronghorn antelope, badgers, and black-footed ferrets. In 1997 he created the Turner Endangered Species Fund to back his belief that he should be "using our good fortune to minimize pain and suffering of others, including other species."

It's important, he says, to set your goals so high you can never achieve them in your lifetime. Turner is a genuine visionary, and he deserves more accolades and recognition from the leaders of the sustainable food movement. He is a fierce proponent of the triple bottom line, which looks beyond the dollars on the balance sheet toward protection of the environment and the benefits to the local and larger community. He has always spoken his mind, and has even publicly admonished fellow billionaires who he thinks should be more generous with their money. Turner backed up his demands by once donating $1 billion to United Nations programs.

As we work to fix our food system and the planet, it's important to hold ourselves to the highest standards, which will truly help future generations live better, more sustainable lives. As Turner likes to say, it's the bottom of the seventh inning and we are down by two runs—it's time to act.

CHAPTER 41

Alphabet Soup

The day is coming when a single carrot, freshly
observed, will set off a revolution.
— *Paul Cézanne*

Behind food and gastronomy exists a myriad of disciplines,
including biology, botany, genetics, physics, chemistry,
agriculture, agronomy, ecology, anthropology, sociology,
economics, politics, technology, history, physiology, nutrition, and medicine. From the first Thanksgiving to the rise
of McDonald's, from the first Native American farmers to
Clarence Birdseye's flash-freezing, from Chef Boyardee and
the men behind Coca-Cola to the great ranchers of Texas
and the cheese makers of Vermont, food defines our
day-to-day existence. It is the ground zero of our success as
a species. Everything in the history of the world — from the
first hunter-gatherers to the Last Supper to sustainable
space travel — can be seen through the lens of food.

It's astonishing that this is somehow lost on American culture. We just don't think about food in a thoughtful, comprehensive way. Look at food media — it's a fashion show. You have to go to the business section or watch a documentary to see coverage of any serious food issue.

We began the Heritage Radio Network to change this, broadcasting from a studio built out of two recycled shipping containers, and even as we grew to thirty-plus shows and three million listeners a month, our spirit remains one of exuberant anarchy. We are making up the rules as we go along.

Breaking down the walls of food complacency need not be so subversive — for all our success broadcasting the gospel from our Brooklyn studio, we recognize that change must come from within the mainstream.

Alice Waters is at the vanguard of food education, a tireless advocate for nothing less than turning lunch period into a hands-on class, like gym or science. There is no American family who would not feel the positive impact if food education became part of the accepted curriculum.

And soon food will have a museum, a physical place, where food culture and history will get the respect they deserve. After all, there are museums for wild animals — the big blue whale and the Hall of African Mammals at New York's American Museum of Natural History are etched into the brains of every kid who has ever been there on a class trip — as well as museums for stamps, medical devices, and balls of twine. Pirates have a museum in Key West, and a voodoo museum exists in New Orleans. There are museums for torture, funeral customs, and pinball machines. Even Burt Reynolds has his own museum.

Individual foods have niche and kitsch museums in their honor—like nuts and vinegars and even Jell-O—but there is not one for food as a whole, in the spirit of the Museum of Science and Industry in Chicago. It's clear that if food is ever going to be elevated in the national consciousness above cooking shows and chef competitions, it needs and deserves a major national brick-and-mortar museum, a destination for school groups, tourists, foodies, a museum as commanding and illuminating as the National Air and Space Museum in DC or the National Baseball Hall of Fame and Museum in Cooperstown.

Thankfully, that is about to come to pass. Our friend Dave Arnold is the prime mover of what will be a temple of food education, the Museum of Food and Drink, or MOFAD. Dave is the founder of the Department of Culinary Technology at the French Culinary Institute (now the International Culinary Center) and the owner of a high-tech cocktail bar called Booker and Dax in New York City. He is also the host of the Heritage Radio Network's *Cooking Issues,* our highest-rated show. In 2004 Dave and the late Michael Batterberry—the founder of *Food & Wine* magazine and *Food Arts* and an American culinary titan on par with James Beard and Julia Child—were talking about the need for a museum dedicated to food. Fast-forward to 2014 and it's finally starting to happen, and I am honored to be on the board of directors.

The American public needs somewhere to go to learn the stories behind what feeds us—whether it's the flow of coffee from around the world to your coffee shop, and how caffeine actually works; or what's really behind the two billion boxes of breakfast cereal consumed in the US every year; or the stories behind digestion, decomposition, dieting, southern food traditions, the spice trade, and how we will eat in the future. MOFAD will be a testament to American agriculture and innovation, an interactive palace where food can be tasted, touched, and seen—a giant leap for mankind.

CHAPTER 42

Don't Be a Hipster Hater

I passionately hate the idea of being with it; I think an artist has always to be out of step with his time.

— *Orson Welles*

Every new subculture was ridiculed at the outset: beatniks, hippies, punk rockers, you name it. And now *hipster* has been hyperventilated as a pejorative so frequently that the word means virtually nothing.

Few movements have suffered as much postmodern shaming as the hippies, but don't forget that in 1968 pretty much everyone with a conscience was one, in some shape or form. There were flower-power hippies and radical hippies. Hippies who went to work and had families, and smelly hippies who turned Haight-Ashbury into an open-air homeless shelter. There was Tiny Tim, and then there was Jimi Hendrix. The Beatles were hippies. The Clintons protested the war in Vietnam—and later lived in the White House. There are lazy hippies, and then there are the hippies who started Apple computers.

What the so-called hipsters aspire to at the most basic level, like the hippies, like the Beats, and like the punks (if we may be so reductive), is what we all should aspire to: breaking away from the status quo. Throwing off the shackles of conformity. Pissing off the squares.

Most poignantly, and closest to the beating heart of THE CARNIVORE'S MANIFESTO, the so-called hipsters have made a massive, positive impact on food culture. They've actualized the highest levels of gastronomy without the white tablecloths: food trucks, barbecue shacks, shops specializing in fresh jams and pickles, bars perpetrating sublime cocktails handcrafted from homemade ingredients, mind-altering pork buns made on a tiny grill.

Unfortunately, snobbery and bias abound. These days, every time someone says "artisanal," half the people in the room roll their eyes. *Artisanal* has become the unfortunate meme of antihipster sarcasm and the curmudgeonly trope of anyone who claims to remember Brooklyn, or Portland— or any number of places where young people have formed a community—before the hipster deluge. But isn't better... *better?*

It would seem that every culture has problems with the one following it (and the one preceding it, for that matter), and to be sure, there are the faux-bohemian poseurs who buy their completely inauthentic version of alternative culture off the rack. But we're saving our vitriol for the people who are really hurting the planet.

Recently, I was looking to get an extended line of credit for Heritage Foods and had little trouble getting approved. The banker told me, "Ya know, ten years ago this would never have gotten through. But right now, young guys in Brooklyn, this progressive food movement, this is a good investment, this is where we want to be." He got it.

CHAPTER 43

I Am a Cow

I never said all actors are cattle; what I said was all actors should be treated like cattle.

—*Alfred Hitchcock*

Good day, friend. Thank you for letting me into your home! If it's all right with you, perhaps we can talk? I promise to be far more civilized than that *awful* ruffian goat. And by the way, the pig isn't the only one in this marvelous book who has been on the cover of a Pink Floyd record. I'm very proud of that.

But more importantly, I'm quite troubled—*vexed*, even!—and want you to understand me. I never asked to eat corn. Not once! Why would I? I am a ruminant—I like to graze. Grass is my thing. My body isn't even built to eat corn. As the calves like to say, "Don't hate the player, hate the game."

McDonald's does not represent me. I am embarrassed

by what they put between their buns. And the "beef" in a Taco Bell taco? I am seriously considering legal action for smearing my good name. The hormones, antibiotics, early weaning, mediocre taste—it is enough to make me weep.

Cows are kind and humble. We have practically no natural enemies. We understand that our popularity in America is based on your love for us—we love you, too! We're proud to be at the center of your cuisine and are well chuffed that you value us so highly as to build restaurants in our honor!

But do you have any idea where I come from? My noble heritage? My lineage is one of honor and fascination—My Ancient White Park cousins were so loved and cherished that Winston Churchill sent a breeding pair to the Toronto Zoo during the war to protect them! A real king—James I —actually knighted the loin section of a White Park, and that's how we came to call it Sir Loin!

Have you heard of the Akaushi? They are the Japanese "Red Cattle," and considered a national treasure! So much are they loved that the Japanese people have agreed to let them roam the sacred mountain of Aso, where they are protected by the government! When three bulls and eight cows left Japan for Texas so Americans could appreciate these noble beasts, they were flown in the kind of airplane that Led Zeppelin used to tour in—they had an armed security detail and were pampered for the entire trip, and then pampered even more as they grazed in their new American home.

We have hundreds of wonderful breeds, and each one is a gastronomic epiphany in its own right. Every hill in Europe has a different genetic line! In France, they know! In South America, they know! We get treated pretty good in Argentina, I hear. In America, mostly we get the McTreatment. And that's why cows everywhere endorse the CARNIVORE'S MANIFESTO.

CHAPTER 44

Slow Business, Part II: How to Make Bread

An investment in knowledge pays the best interest.
—*Benjamin Franklin*

Alice Waters told me the story of a wonderful business in the food world that serves as a great model for any organization that wants to expand without losing its soul. It's the formula for growing without having to centralize all the power on top of a mountain, without having to neuter workers or strip the personal touch from the product.

Pierre Poilâne opened a bakery in France in 1932 at 8 rue du Cherche-Midi in Paris's Saint-Germain-des-Prés district. At the time, Poilâne Bakery was the smallest of the five bakeries on the street, though eighty-two years later it is the only one still in operation. You may have heard of him—Poilâne is now among the most revered names in bread on the planet.

Pierre founded his bakery on the timelessness of what we call *le têtoir boulanger,* and his bakery thrived. It probably didn't hurt that he became beloved as much for his love of Paris and his sense of community as for his bread—he was known to trade bread for paintings by local artists.

When Pierre suffered a stroke in 1973, his son Lionel took over. Lionel opened more bakeries in Paris, and one in London, and also became a potent ambassador for his bread, and the Frenchness of bread itself, which is something you cannot fake. No shucking and jiving—if it hadn't been authentic he could have been the first head to roll off the guillotine in years.

He also understood the value of art and artisanship. He built the world's largest library of books about bread and bread making, studying every known regional variety. In a lighter mood, he built a bedroom for Salvador Dalí out of dough.

Under Lionel, Poilâne expanded its volume significantly, but cautiously, never relying on cheap, mass-produced baked goods spewed out on a conveyor belt or turning its employees into automatons with little input into the final product.

In 1981 Poilâne opened a new production facility in Bièvre, which is just outside Paris. And this is where Lionel implemented a concept he called retro-innovation, a combination of traditional principles and creative solutions that met the current realities and expectations of Poilâne's markets. He had figured out how to do big business and still deliver a handcrafted *miche*—Poilâne's signature wheel of sourdough bread.

Lionel organized the baking teams on the production floor of his new "manufactory" in a sun-ray pattern emanating from a pile of dry cherry wood that stood in the center of the room. Every section was managed by an independent baking team, which orchestrated its production schedule and worked as if it were an independent bakery. Which effectively meant that on a roster of, say, one hundred bakers, no one was at the bottom of the pecking order—you came in no lower than number five on a team made up of your partners in excellence.

Lionel also implemented a strict system of quality assessment at the Bièvre bakery. One representative loaf of every batch, identified by the first name of the head baker, was placed on a tray cart and presented for inspection. The loaves were then closely examined, sliced, smelled, and tested for their pH levels.

Every man or woman on that floor had the dignity and pride that comes with having a hand in a great tradition, so grand that *The New Yorker* called it "bread's most venerable brand, the Louis Vuitton of boulangers," although bread is one of those magic things that transcends social class. The product never lost the rural notes of the unpolished, Old

World technique that Parisians understood as integral to true French bread. Poilâne didn't even use thermometers.

Currently, according to a *New Yorker* profile on the bakery, under Pierre's granddaughter Apollonia, Poilâne grosses $18 million a year and has more than 150 employees, many of whom spend their entire careers there. They take pride in everything that comes out of that oven — every loaf stamped with the *P* for *Poilâne*. Their boss has never forgotten that the fine line of art and craft is usually drawn with the charming inconsistencies of the handmade.

CHAPTER 45

It's the Meat

Heaven sends us good meat, but the Devil sends cooks.

—*David Garrick*

Want a hot recipe? Here's one: Choose a lovely, well-sourced piece of meat—from a merchant you trust, from a farm you know, and from a breed you have come to love, and add fire. *Et voilà!* There's your recipe. Just remember, the fire is the constant, the meat is the variable. And don't forget where it came from, so you can do it again.

Cooking is easy. Mother Nature + the skill of a responsible farmer = the only recipe you should ever fuss over. Rather than filling your shelves with epic recipe books, how about breed charts that describe the gastronomic wonders of every livestock variety? "One 32-ounce flank steak" as the prime mover in a recipe is not enough information for the enlightened carnivore. Where does that beef come from—farm and breed, please! And was it from a happy cow that led a decent cow life grazing and doing happy cow things? Or was it a prisoner of American industry?

Cattle are a lot more nuanced than you might think. Dig this: Piedmontese and Belgian Blues are the only two breeds of cow that have the "double-muscle" gene, which makes them extraordinarily tender. And these cows are loaded with myostatin, a protein that inhibits muscle differentiation and growth. As a result, you get a supremely tender and delicious cut of beef. Contrast that with the Angus—which has more tooth and is especially good for dry-aging. The Simmental, a Swiss cow originally bred to stand up to thin air in the Alps, requires a serious knife and some sharp incisors when it comes time to eating. But its grain packs a lot of distinct flavor.

Turning to pigs, the Gloucestershire Old Spot is so sweet and creamy, tucking into one of its chops is like having a glass of buttermilk. And our old friend the Red Wattle is what I would call superpork—its taste is mega-swiney and powerful! The Tamworth pig is something else entirely—it's a lean breed that doesn't deliver the sweet smack of the fat, but you get a more refined taste that practically screams for a dollop of applesauce. But that's it, a dollop, because the breed is where the excitement comes from, not the mélange of shmancy flavors you paint it with. Asphyxiating meat with spices and waterboarding it with sauce is just this side of animal cruelty. At best all you are doing is covering up for mediocre meat, which you shouldn't be buying or eating in the first place.

The Katahdin lamb is a hair sheep, rather than a wool sheep, so it's low in lanolin, giving it a very mild taste. Other breeds, like Black Welsh Mountain, have a powerful lamby taste. Different occasions cry for different breeds—and the same goes for turkeys, ducks, chickens, geese, you name it.

Carnivores should know their favorite beasts as well as New Yorkers know the subway map—if New York were a cow, perhaps Fifth Avenue would be the strip steak and Times Square the brisket, and wouldn't it be a tragedy not to understand what each has to offer? As Walt Whitman once said, "I have traveled greatly in Manhattan." San Francisco would of course be a different kind of cow, with varied flavors and textures, some earthier, some more flamboyant.

Being intimate with the supply chain is where it's at, which is why THE CARNIVORE'S MANIFESTO is an ingredient-based philosophy. Be a friend and fan of the beast. Food is very personal, and knowledge is power. And when it comes right down to it, it's the meat, not the motion.

CHAPTER 46

Splendor in the Tallgrass

A nation that destroys its soils destroys itself.
— *Franklin Delano Roosevelt*

It is hard to say which *terroir* in America produces the best beef. Some would argue for the Willamette Valley in Oregon, which spans from Eugene to Portland, one of the grassiest and most fertile spots in the country. Others would argue that the hot summers and mild-to-cool winters make Georgia the perfect place for cattle to grow up pampered and stress free, while the hillsides and grassy valleys of the Finger Lakes certainly make for some very happy cows. Texas, Colorado, and Montana might have something to say about it as well.

But for THE CARNIVORE'S MANIFESTO, the best *terroir* for beef is the Flint Hills—a band of hills that stretches from eastern Kansas into north-central Oklahoma, extending from Marshall and Washington Counties in Kansas in the

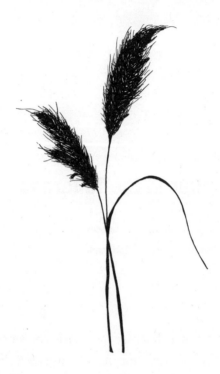

north, to Cowley County in Kansas and Kay and Osage Counties in Oklahoma in the south.

Anywhere tallgrass grows makes for a great and sustainable *terroir* for cattle, but what makes the Flint Hills our number-one choice is that it boasts the most dense coverage of intact tallgrass prairie in North America and has blossomed into a mosaic of independent family farms—many of which are at the heart of the heritage breed movement.

Tallgrass is the food the prairie produces naturally in the absence of intensive row-crop agriculture. Unlike corn, tallgrass is not dependent on petrochemical fertilizer or herbicide, and its roots run deep below the thin layer of top-soil. It is potent, incredibly resilient, the all-you-can-eat salad bar for healthy cattle. And they love it, gladly eating twenty pounds of the stuff every day. Cows are ruminants, meaning they were built to consume grass and not grain, which they are fed on almost all industrial farms.

The result of this robust food supply is a steak with a nice even ratio of intra- and extramuscular fat, a beefy and clean taste, perhaps not as buttery as the corn-fed cattle we've gotten used to, but more finely nuanced, a natural delight. It is the taste of the Americas.

Varietals like Bluestem, Little Bluestem, Indiangrass, Switchgrass, Prairie Dropseed, and Sideoats Grama have stalks whose profound roots are able to pull moisture and nutrients from deep within the ground, making them the best candidates to withstand the drought and deluge likely to accompany climate change. They are resistant to all types of extreme weather, and they bounce back quickly, even from fires. And they do not rely on the dwindling power of the thin layer of topsoil to grow.

Wes Jackson of the Land Institute in Salina, Kansas, has been a major spokesperson in defense of soil and in promo-tion of tallgrass, and has been working to develop a new perennial wheat grass, Kernza, that may come to replace the topsoil-depleting annuals. His goal is to feed the world when agriculture fails us, which it will one day. If we restored just a portion of the Corn Belt to the tallgrass prai-rie it once was, and got back to using it as pasture for cattle to graze on—free-ranging animals aerate and nourish the land—it would go a long way toward stopping soil erosion, the poisonous nitrogen runoff that causes ecological dead zones, and the corn industry's vampirelike addiction to fossil fuel.

THE CARNIVORE'S MANIFESTO calls for the Industrial Food Complex—including McDonald's, Cargill, and anyone responsible for raising or selling mass-produced corn-fed beef—to begin the slow turning of the wheel to restore some type of "permaculture" to the terrain, and commit to a long-term goal of significantly reducing the footprint of damaging, nonsustainable agriculture. They owe it to the planet they are beating up, as well as to their shareholders—not to mention the cows.

CHAPTER 47

Letter to a Farmer

Farming is a profession of hope.
　　—Brian Brett

Dear Independent American Farmer,

The revolution begins in your backyard. From the smallest burger grill to the bumper crop of chef-driven restaurants, the demand for food that is as sustainable as it is delicious gets bigger every day. And as more people consider starting farms, and as existing farms steer their businesses toward more responsible practices, I'd like to share with you some of the things I've learned from my farmer friends as we've worked together over the last fifteen years.

Differentiate. Grow or raise a unique product—an exclusive breed or heirloom seed. By any means necessary, you must differentiate yourself from the lowest common denominator of just pumping out more-of-the-same chops or growing beautiful but undistinguished tomatoes. The market is there for quality, and it will reward your ingenuity and differentiation. This is the key to busting free from the grip of commodity culture and its oppressive, nonsustainable price points.

Quality includes customer service and delivery times. Anything less than a 98 percent delivery success rate is a sign of impending failure. Don't ever overpromise on weight of carcass or number of units. Don't send something different than what is ordered and hope your customer will make an exception. If you don't take your business seriously, no one else will. If you fuck up, give a refund, and then some. Nothing is more important than the customer.

Work in numbers. Invest in communal enterprises with like-minded individuals. In Europe, it is far more common for small farmers to work in co-ops, and the result is more business for everyone. Sharing infrastructure will make you stronger—whether it's a better delivery van or sharing a driver, or renting a refrigerated warehouse, or building a slaughterhouse—enjoy the economy of scale. Sharing improves your standing and gravitas. You'll have backups and contingencies. Be fiercely aggressive about partnering, but remember, one bad farmer can ruin it for the rest. Shun him, for he will make a desert of his home and yours. He is the harbinger of death.

Avoid fool's gold. When somebody tells you they sold a pork tenderloin for $80 a pound, or squeals that they found a ten-pound truffle out by the old elm tree, don't think it is going to happen to you. Don't use miracles as the foundation of your business. And don't use the Union Square Greenmarket in New York City as your model—they sell to some of the most affluent gourmands in America! Look to the farmers' markets on the outskirts of town to find a more realistic rubric.

Befriend the sad reality of the loss leader. —And it needs to be something good. On the pig, the loin is the most cherished cut, and at Heritage Meat Shop we sell our loin chops for $8 a pound, the best deal in New York City. We don't make the margin we could, but it breeds loyalty. It's our ambassador to potential converts who just need to taste our meats once to become fans. I can't even imagine how many discounted chops turned into big sales of steaks and charcuterie, whole goats and lambs.

You need a low-end wholesale outlet. When an account falls through, and it will happen, selling off your inventory for cheap is a lot better than seeing a stockpile of bellies build up in your freezers. The wholesale market, and sadly the commodity market, too, is like the morning-after pill for the meat business. It's insurance. When you need an out, it helps you sleep at night, even if it breaks your heart that your pristine products might end up in supermarket sausages. And know, too, which restaurants you can sell to at fire-sale prices—the trick is to know when to pull the trigger. Farms always need to prepare for the worst. That's the business.

Beware of value-added products. This could be just more fool's gold—a value-added product is not the same as the product itself. Just because you grow fantastic blackberries doesn't mean you can make fantastic blackberry jam. Being a great pig farmer doesn't make you an ace sausage maker. But if you can do it right, or partner with someone who can, it can be the road to more profit. A fresh ham sells for $2 a pound. A cured one for $10.

Beware of the false promises of mail order. I can't tell you how many times I've heard a farmer say that his Internet site was going to be the tipping point in his business. Take it from me: Mail order is a pain in the ass—it's time-consuming, you need thousands of potential customers on a list just to sell to a few, you have to navigate the vagaries of shipping and jockey for a discount with FedEx or UPS, and it is absolutely impossible to predict what a person at home is going to order over the Internet, no matter how good you think your e-mail list is.

Never advertise. All good things rely on word of mouth, and never paid advertising or spin.

> *The number of people out there who are looking for high-quality, sustainable, fair food is growing every day. Nobody works harder than you, and as traditional agricultural values take fresh root, we wish you only the best, and pledge our continued support—nothing would be better for America than to see more good farms producing more good food.*
>
> *Sincerely,*
>
> THE CARNIVORE'S MANIFESTO

CHAPTER 48

Don't Forget to Feast

Dost thou think, because thou art virtuous, there
shall be no more cakes and ale?
— *William Shakespeare,* Twelfth Night

Even the most Dickensian of us, Charles Dickens himself,
knew that "vices are sometimes only virtues carried to
excess." And so I ask you, What happened to the feast?
Feasts for the saints! Feasts to honor the gods! Old-school
medieval banquets so indulgent that they could level an
entire city-state!

I'm not talking about forty-ounce Big Gulps or hundred-
piece buckets of chicken, Supersized Value Meals, or two-
fer pizzas with a box of bread and a bucket of cheese
product. That's just gross and sad, empty calories filing
empty lives. I'm talking about Blake's road to wisdom,
paved in excess! And I'm addressing *you,* dear reader, the

supposedly enlightened and literate lover of food, and I am challenging you to come with me into gastronomic overdrive. I am talking about the romanticizing not just of food, but of *eating*. In the words of Mae West, later purloined so wonderfully by the king of conspicuous consumption, Liberace, "Too much of a good thing can be wonderful!"

I'm just like everyone else who has crossed over the demarcation line into their get-fat forties. I have to keep an eye on my figure or no one else will. And so I don't eat five-thousand-calorie lunches every day. But I still find time for the unhinged celebration at Fort Defiance—oysters! An aged steak with a Matterhorn of *frites!* Zingy cocktails, thoughtful wine, and a broadside of a dessert before the knock-down *digestif!*

Once upon a time, America was populated by religious groups who couldn't get along with anybody in Europe because they were just too goddamn severe about everything. That energy still persists, and even today, even as we gobble double cheeseburgers and guzzle Big Gulps, we fear pleasure as if it were evil. This is a country that lives in fear of sin—sex and gluttony are at the top of the list—while simultaneously running toward it. It's a complex relationship that builds walls between us and our pleasure centers. Sometimes we just need to let go.

We need to allow food its full potential to be realized as a gorgeous pleasure, and not handed out like rare jewels, as with nickel-sized medallions of veal that look large only in comparison to the lonely wisp of greens or the parsimonious ejaculation of whipped root vegetables that make up their dying bed.

We aren't advocating for lumberjack breakfasts seven days a week, nor endless racks of ribs with all the fixin's and pecan pie every night of the week. Hasn't Paula Deen already created enough trouble? But foie gras, biscuits and gravy, cured meats, and copious spirits are as much part of a sustainable diet as are rice cakes and chia seeds.

As in all things, of course, a little common sense could prevail. Remember well the words of Somerset Maugham, who said, "Excess on occasion is exhilarating. It prevents moderation from acquiring the deadening effect of a habit."

I'm sick of hearing about how many calories I should consume if I don't want to be hauled off to fat camp and shunned by the general population. I'm sick of people telling me to eat only plants. Sure, health is wealth and all we want is for everyone to live a long life, but we also need to have times of wild abandon.

In the Middle Ages, feasts happened when food was abundant: the festivals of spring, summer, and fall. Feasting was a way of allowing yourself a temporary respite from your troubles, sometimes to a point bordering on revolution—during Carnival, kings behaved as paupers in a complete inversion of society, while the proles ruled the roost. The idea was, better to go all out tonight because you never know what tomorrow will bring. As Bill Hicks once said, "If you live for tomorrow you will always be a day late."

Carnival is a time of intense laughter and regeneration,

a time to fight back against our culture of denial and guilt. Acting out is important, because, as my esteemed and wise coauthor likes to say, "A little bit of crazy keeps the big crazy away."

I eat healthy, responsible food. Mostly. But sometimes I want to go one toke over the line. I'm talking about Rabelais, and Gargantua. Now, that dude knew how to eat! I'm taking a page from his book, and one from Oscar Wilde's, who would like to remind us that "Moderation is a fatal thing. Nothing succeeds like excess," and, even more importantly, "Where there is no extravagance there is no love, and where there is no love there is no understanding."

So for dinner tonight I think I'll order two hundred portions of grilled octopus shipped in from Spain, drizzled with olive oil from Sicily, and gilded with a few grains of sea salt from off the coast of Portugal.

Once my appetite is piqued, I'll dig into a plate of *carne cruda,* a ball of raw meat no smaller than a watermelon. It's better than steak tartare, prepared with olive oil and lemon instead of a cracked egg so it's that much lighter. See? I am very sensible about these things.

For the next round, more meat, of course, but nothing too heavy, as I am still just prepping my incisors for the main event. Perhaps just thirty or forty appetizer-sized portions of Akaushi eye of round carpaccio, served with a delicate Parmigiano-Reggiano, aged for exactly two years, no more and no less, to give the whole thing some legs and help it dance on my palate.

Clearly, I'm going to need some wine to wash this down with — I think we'll start with some Bandol Tempier. Two cases should be just fine, it is so easy to drink! And then something a little bigger, perhaps a Barbaresco. Along with sparkling water, I am thinking a few cases of Budweiser — it really does go with anything.

While waiting for the main course I always like to amuse myself, and I think, in this case, a half dozen or so of New York City's greatest gastronomic gift to the world of noshing ought to do it: the everything bagel with lox. And of course, wild Alaskan salmon is the only salmon that can stand up to a bagel covered in seeds, red onions, capers, and cream cheese.

And now I am ready to rumble.

For the main course, a bit of Eastern flair would be a good turn: two dozen Pekin ducks from Good Shepherd Ranch in Lindsborg, Kansas, prepared Peking style with pancakes and plum sauce and scallions, which I'll roll up like fat, duck-filled doobies and wash down with a dark beer from North Coast Brewing Company that is just bitter enough to groove with the sweet meat and not fight it.

Just to prove to everyone that I am not crazy, this will be the time for something green. Three Caesar salads will do, prepared tableside, and don't be stingy with the ancho-vies, preferably from SeaLab Italia, in Bra. Now the way is clear for the cheese course, which I prefer in the form of a hot tub of fondue of raw-milk cheeses from my favorite

East Coast dairies—Meadow Creek Dairy, Spring Brook Farm, and Landaff Creamery.

For dessert, a baker's dozen of *quindim pies*—a custardy Brazilian delicacy that is so time intensive to make, what with its hundred-eggs-per-pie mandate, that hardly anyone besides my mom makes it anymore. She whipped one up for me last year for Independence Day—you would know it by the trail of comatose bodies it left in its wake.

But before I call it a night, I'll take my time with three bottles of Fernet Branca. No matter how popular it gets with the trend chasers, it's still the one thing I can count on to help calm the ol' gullet after a snack like the one I just imagined. It's kind of like Jägermeister for adults.

CHAPTER 49

A Fairy Tale

Imagination is more important than knowledge.

—*Albert Einstein*

Once upon a time there was a small, peaceful village filled with cheerful people.

The village had a Main Street lined with shops run by shopkeepers. There was a butcher who cut meat, a cobbler who made shoes, a baker who baked bread, a tailor who made clothes, and a toymaker who made the most magical toys. In the town square there was a café where all the townspeople would drink coffee, read their newspapers, and talk to one another.

One morning a man no one had ever seen before rode into town with a horse and cart. He was tall and thin as a pencil and wore a stovepipe hat. He had small, dark eyes and a greasy mustache that he twirled between his long, thin fingers.

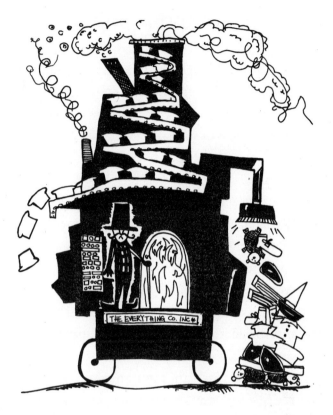

Atop the cart there was a gigantic machine that rose a hundred feet into the air. It had chutes and spouts and fidgets and widgets, and black smoke and dirt spewed out of its smokestack.

The stranger pulled his cart into the middle of the square, and from his perch on top of his horse, he called out to the townspeople. Everyone gathered around to hear what he had to say.

"Good townsfolk, I am the president of the Everything Company and I'm here to make your lives much better!

From now on I can provide all the things you need in life, made by my Everything Machine!"

The stranger pointed to the butcher and said, "No longer will your hand hurt from sharpening your knives and cutting meat. And you, cobbler, my Everything Machine can make fifty pairs of shoes an hour! Just think of all the things you can do if you don't have to make shoes all day." To the baker he said, "Now you can sleep until noon and never have to wake up early to bake bread again. Tailor, imagine what my machine can do for clothes. All you have to do is put cloth in one side, push a button, and out the other come dresses, pants, and shirts in any color or shape or size your heart desires. Toymaker, enough with your silly painted wooden toys! My Everything Machine can make any toy in the world out of my patented plastic Gobbledygook!"

"Could this be true?" the townspeople asked. "No need to stand in line and wait for the meat to be cut or the bread to be baked, no need to wait two weeks for a toy to be ready or shoes to be repaired?" They all agreed it was an interesting proposition indeed.

The shopkeepers thought about what the stranger had said. The baker was the first to speak. "I learned how to bake bread from my father and he from his father. I have been baking bread for thirty years. How can a machine know how to do it better than I?"

Then the cobbler said, "I am an old man. Over the years I have made thousands of shoes for every kind of foot. For the narrowest feet and the fattest feet, for the youngest feet and the oldest. What machine could make a better shoe than I?"

The toymaker asked, "How does the Everything Machine know what the children want? And even if it does, I make the best toys in the land! Could a machine do that?"

The butcher and the tailor agreed. How, they wondered, could a machine that made bread, shoes, and toys also know how to cut meat and sew clothes? It just didn't make sense.

Soon there was a big ruckus and people began to shout. The townsfolk were fascinated by the promises made by the stranger in the black hat, but the shopkeepers were angry to think that their services would no longer be needed after all these years.

The mayor heard the fighting from his office in the town hall. He summoned his deputies and they marched out to the square. "What's going on here?" the mayor roared. "What's happened to my peaceful town?"

The stranger and the shopkeepers made their case. The mayor listened to them carefully, thought it over for a few minutes, and came up with a plan.

"This stranger claims his Everything Machine can make the best of absolutely everything," he called out to the townspeople. "Meanwhile, the shopkeepers claim that their goods are the finest money can buy. There's only one way to settle this fairly and squarely—I hereby declare a contest between the Everything Machine and the shopkeepers! Both shall work from sunrise to sundown, making the very best of the things they make. At the end of the day, the townspeople will decide who goes and who stays."

It was decided that the contest would take place the very next day.

As the cobbler walked home that night, his lip quivered at the thought of losing his shop. And the tailor wondered how he would spend his days if he couldn't make the clothes that filled his imagination day and night. The toymaker's eyes welled up with tears at the thought of never again seeing the happy faces of the children who so loved his toys. The baker and the butcher did not sleep a wink that night, wondering what their families would do if the Everything Machine won. The stranger just slept soundly in his cart.

Before the sun rose, the square was bursting with people. The farmers marched in from the fields, the fishermen docked their boats, the teachers and the principal locked the school door and came with all the schoolchildren in tow. The shopkeepers' families and friends crowded around to whoop and cheer them on. Even the town's dogs and cats came to see what all the hoopla was about. Never before had the town square held so many people all at one time.

The shopkeepers lined up across one side of the square. There was a long wooden table for them to work on, and each had a station. The butcher sharpened her meat cleaver. The toymaker gathered the wood and lined up his pots of paint and brushes. The baker fed logs into his oven, and the cobbler got out his best leather and his favorite hammer. The tailor took out his strongest needle and thread.

Meanwhile, on the other side of the square, the stranger sat alongside the Everything Machine in a plush chair, pushing different buttons and calmly puffing on his pipe. The Everything Machine huffed and puffed and sputtered and spouted. When the sun rose above the horizon, the mayor yelled out, "Let the competition begin!"

The baker's face soon turned red as a beet from the heat of the fire. His hands and arms felt as heavy as lead from carrying heavy bags of flour and kneading his loaves of bread. He toiled harder than anyone had ever seen him toil before, and as the hours passed, a small pile, then a large hill, and then a veritable mountain of bread formed by the side of his oven.

The cobbler rolled out the finest blue leather that anyone had ever seen. It was made from the softest cowhide and was dyed brilliant blue with the juice of ten thousand blueberries. He cut and shaped the leather and then painstakingly nailed the soles to the bottoms of the shoes, using a hundred nails that were so small that only a few people could see them, much less hold them in position and hit their heads with a hammer.

The toymaker's fingers started to ache as he tinkered and assembled and painted and glued. Children crowded around and jumped and cheered as he set rocking horses rocking, colored balls bouncing, and train sets choo-chooing.

He always liked to say, "My tops are the top—just one turn and they'll spin for days!" Legend had it that one of his tops had once spun for four days straight.

The tailor threaded his needle and sewed so quickly that his fingers became a blur. His motto was "Never a glitch with nary a stitch!" and today was no different. Rainbows of thread spun off their spools as he whirled and swirled around his mannequins, crafting beautiful costumes for men and women of all shapes and sizes.

The butcher's knife glimmered and gleamed in the sun as she cleaved and cut perfectly portioned steaks, stuffed a bajillion sausages, skewered succulent kebabs, and made three perfect pyramids of pâté.

Meanwhile, the Everything Machine chugged and churned away as humungous clouds of smoke spewed out of its top. All the shoes and steaks and toys and shirts and bread shot out of the same pipe and landed in neat piles around the town square.

The sun was about to set and the shopkeepers were exhausted—their hands hurt and so did their backs and feet and arms and legs. They had each sweated through five sets of shirts and aprons. At one point, the toymaker almost gave up. But when he saw the children staring at him with their wide and hopeful eyes, he felt a final burst of energy and put the finishing touches on three teddy bears and four bouncy balls. The shopkeepers continued working almost as fast as when the competition had begun, until the last ray of sun dipped out of sight.

Finally, the church bell rang, signaling the end of the competition.

All the goods produced that day were lined up on the long wooden table and presented to the people for judgment.

First, the townspeople bit into the loaves of bread. The loaves the baker had baked were heavenly: crusty and airy and warm and delicious. As they crunched and munched and chewed and chawed, they felt happiness from their teeth to their taste buds to the bottoms of their bellies!

Every loaf that came out of the Everything Machine looked very tasty, too. But when the people picked one up to take a bite, they realized that something was wrong. It looked like bread, and it smelled like bread, but it was missing *something*. They couldn't figure out quite what it was, but they soon lost interest in the Everything Machine's bread and demanded more loaves from the baker.

Next they tried on the clothes. The shirts, pants, and dresses that had come out of the Everything Machine looked superb. But when the townsfolk put them on, they didn't quite fit. The fabric stretched, the seams ripped, and when they tried to move, some of the buttons popped off, leaving the ladies and gentlemen in their underwear. The crowd shrieked as their faces turned red.

The clothing the tailor had made and the shoes the cobbler had cobbled were sturdy and beautiful and made to last for many years. The women who wore what was produced that day looked so stunning that it took everyone's breath away. Young men rushed in and kneeled at their feet, asking for their hands in marriage. They had never seen such beauty before!

Next the children came out from behind the grown-ups to inspect the toys. They ran up to the shiny pile that the Everything Machine had made, squealing with delight. There were rocket ships and dump trucks and jump ropes and grandiose thingamajigs! But soon after the children picked up the toys to play with them, their faces fell. It was hard for the children to describe just what was wrong, but there was no magic in these toys—despite all their bells and whistles and switches and sparkles, the Everything toys were ho-hum.

The children started to cry, but then the toymaker called out to them. They ran to him, marveling at the wooden rocking horses with their beautiful painted manes and the spinning tops that never stopped and the choo-choo trains that puffed around tracks across the square. Each and every toy had so much magic in it that as soon as the children picked one up, they began to laugh and clap their hands with joy.

While the children skipped and jumped about with glee, the grow-ups moved in to judge the meats. The steaks and sausages made by the Everything Machine looked mouthwatering. But when the townsfolk cut into them with their knives and forks, they were surprised to find bits of buttons, strings of thread, and globs of Gobbledygook inside. "Eeek!" they all cried. "Your Everything steaks are full of leftover bits and pieces of all the shoes and toys and clothes and loaves of terrible bread!" Even the dogs and cats in attendance took one sniff and ran the other way.

Then the people turned to their trusted butcher, mouths watering. She had prepared an enormous feast, and the townsfolk dug right in, savoring her perfect steaks, succulent sausages, killer kebabs, and princely pâtés. They finished every last bite, wiping their lips with napkins and sighing with delight.

The decision was unanimous. The shopkeepers had won, no ifs, ands, or buts!

The townsfolk glared menacingly across the square at the stranger, who had already hitched his Everything Machine to his horse, which he was kicking in a tizzy as he tried to flee.

The townsfolk began to cheer. They shook the shopkeepers' hands, lifted them onto their shoulders, and paraded them around the square. And they apologized for ever having doubted them.

They shouted at the stranger, "Get out of here with your Everything Machine! We have everything we need here, and much better things than your silly machine could ever make!"

Just then, the stranger's horse broke into a gallop, but the wheels of the cart began to quiver and creak. In an instant they gave out, and the Everything Machine crashed to the ground with a thunderous thump. It puttered and sputtered and then it was still.

The stranger unhitched his cart, kicked his horse, and

rode away, leaving the Everything Machine broken down in the town square.

Today, when people visit the town, the gargantuan remains of the Everything Machine still sit there, but its smokestacks are planted with beautiful flowers and vines, and its sides are covered with beautiful scenes painted by the town's children. It sits there as a reminder to the towns-folk to always trust the slow and steady hand of the artisan.

CHAPTER 50

In the Year 2222...

Food Culture has become as important a part of the curriculum in American schools as reading, writing, and arithmetic, and a high school cafeteria in the Bronx is the first to be awarded a Michelin star.

The cost of high-fructose corn syrup skyrockets following the Permaculture Act of 2221, which helps turn America's Corn Belt into grazing land for cattle.

After a massive federal bailout fails to save it, McDonald's joins the internal-combustion engine on the scrap heap of history.

National rationing of potable water is averted when Budweiser debuts the first beer made from desalinated seawater.

*   *   *

A superintelligent cow—a mutation caused by excessive antibiotics and hormones—has successfully sued conglomerate agriculture giant Cargill-Tyson in a class-action suit for abuse and willful negligence, and as a condition of the settlement has become the first bovine board member of a publicly traded company.

A strain of genetically modified chickens that grow to be five feet tall and are covered in wings—like roses on a rosebush—are developed by the newly formed bioengineering department of ExxonMobilPerdue, but plans to make them the industry standard backfire when one of the chickens escapes and is videotaped terrorizing a shopping mall in Idaho. In the aftermath, horrified Americans begin to reject factory-farmed chicken, leading Frank Perdue XIV to exclaim to shareholders, "We've just lost Detroit!"

New York's Central Park Zoo makes headlines when it puts on display the last flock of the once-dominant Broad Breasted White turkey, now an endangered species. Meanwhile, the Occupy Sheep Meadow movement has been largely successful in repopulating Central Park's Sheep Meadow with actual sheep.

★　　★　　★

With Lower Manhattan now below sea level, Poughkeepsie becomes the new restaurant capital of America.

Yankee Stadium declares that all food served during ball games will be locally produced and sourced from local farms—except for the mustard.

Poultry overtakes beef as the most expensive meat on the menu, and competitive breeding wars explode in the backyards of Brooklyn, Seattle, and Salt Lake City—the new hipster Mecca—much like the tulip wars in seventeenth-century Holland.

Niche restaurants and markets have blossomed in the most unlikely places—garage cheese makers, bakers, and artisanal cocktail bars pepper suburbia, and a new wave of micro-kitchens turns out pickles and charcuterie from the solar-powered houseboats that now clog the Chesapeake Bay.

Following the Fair Labor Acts of 2020 and 2112, and the Living Wage Act of 2217, empty Walmart buildings have been repurposed as giant greenhouses and botanical gardens.

★   ★   ★

Macy's National Farmers' Day Sale offers tractors in designer colors for fashionable urban farmers.

The 2222 edition of *The Whole Earth Catalog* is the first to be printed entirely on seaweed. It pairs nicely with a dry soju.

Organic goat tacos replace chicken wings as the number-one food served on Super Bowl Sunday. Grass-fed bison chili nachos come in at number two.

The Smithsonian Museum of Marijuana History and Culture opens in Washington, DC, with the president unveiling a hundred-foot statue of Willie Nelson.

The Museum of Food and Drink Gala Bicentennial Ball is held on the new International Space Platform and catered entirely with food grown in space. Meanwhile, the first restaurant to open on Moonbase Alpha specializes in meatballs.

The thirty-eighth edition of THE CARNIVORE'S MANIFESTO is released by Little, Brown. Martins and Edison, its original authors, are long dead and forgotten. Which reminds us: We all end up as dirt, so please, eat well, have fun — and leave the place better than you found it.

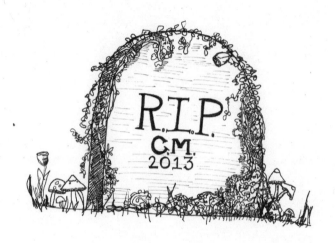

Essential Reading

Alice's Adventures in Wonderland, by Lewis Carroll. If you can navigate this tale, you can change the world.

Animals Make Us Human: Creating the Best Life for Animals, by Temple Grandin and Catherine Johnson. The only book you need to read to learn how to respect all animals the right way.

The Botany of Desire: A Plant's-Eye View of the World, by Michael Pollan. This is still my favorite of Michael's books, and for me one of the best food books ever written.

The Encyclopedia of Historic and Endangered Livestock and Poultry Breeds, by Janet Vorwald Dohner. The encyclopedia every serious meat eater must own.

Gargantua and Pantagruel, by Rabelais. A masterful, wildly hilarious tale of two giants. The eating and drinking scenes remain the funniest ever.

Fast Food Nation: The Dark Side of the All-American Meal, by Eric Schlosser. The essential muckraking food book

of our time. To read this is to never eat at McDonald's
again.

Guns, Germs, and Steel: The Fates of Human Societies, by Jared
Diamond. This is a must-read if you want to understand how almost everything everywhere came to be
the way it is.

*Highbrow/Lowbrow: The Emergence of Cultural Hierarchy in
America,* by Lawrence W. Levine. One of my favorite
books, which taught me that what's lowbrow one
moment can arbitrarily be considered highbrow another.

Hungry City: How Food Shapes Our Lives, by Carolyn Steel. A
great book that uncovers the connection between agriculture and cities.

On the Future of Food, by HRH The Prince of Wales. Prince
Charles shows real courage in talking the way he does
about the Industrial Food Complex. This is a great
speech, and HRH is a great fighter for our cause.

*Physiology of Taste, or Meditations on Transcendental Gastron-
omy,* by Jean Anthelme Brillat-Savarin. You cannot
properly call yourself a gourmand until you have read
this 1825 treatise on taste, eating, cooking, and general
snobbery.

*Slow Food Nation: Why Our Food Should Be Good, Clean and
Fair,* by Carlo Petrini. The best book ever written by
the founder of Slow Food.

Steal This Book, by Abbie Hoffman. A spirited instrument of
anarchy, still an inspiration.

This Organic Life: Confessions of a Suburban Homesteader, by
    Joan Dye Gussow. Joan was leading the cause before
    most people even knew there was a cause.

The Whole Earth Catalog. They printed many editions over
    many years. Go online, get your hands on a copy. And
    participate in the publication of a new edition!

Acknowledgments

Thanks first to my collaborator and friend Mike Edison, who has fueled this book with his energy, wit, and word-smithery. Mike has the patience of Job and the strength of a thousand men. He is a true champion.

I want to thank Renée Gerson for pushing me to travel and to learn new languages. Thanks to Tris and Charles Steinberg, Toby Tumarkin, Brian Kenny, and Dan MacKay for keeping me sane.

Thanks to my professor and friend Barbara Kirshenblatt-Gimblett, who opened my eyes to the potential of the food revolution.

Thanks to my agent (and favorite goat farmer), Angela Miller, for fighting for us and our fifty essays, and to Mike's team at Dystel & Goderich Literary Management.

Thanks to Michael Sand and everyone at Little, Brown for making this book possible.

Heritage Foods USA and Heritage Radio Network are powered by so many great people: Serena Di Liberto has been leading the food fight since 1999 — since before Slow Food came to American shores — and has been the most trustworthy part of every business I've ever been a part of. Erin Fairbanks inspired a food revolution on the airwaves and on goat farms from the moment she arrived off a vegetable truck from Michigan, slung a pig carcass over her shoulder, and started making weekly deliveries.

Catherine Greeley is a font of positive energy and has led our mail-order division (HeritageFoodsUSA.com) to success never before imagined — please order meats from our site and see for yourself! Dick Bessey, Leah Eden, Emile Frohlich, Joe Galarraga, Jack Inslee, Janani Lee, Kieran McShane, and Dionisio Silva fight the good fight every day. Thank you.

Heritage Foods USA exists because of folks like Frank Reese, the greatest poultry breeder in America. Sam Edwards is a friend, a mentor, and a tremendous supporter of our network, thanks to his skills in the high art of charcuterie. Taylor and Toponia Boetticher have created an empire of cured meats around the Bay Area that is also an anchor for our network. Mark Ladner, Zach Allen, and Mario Batali and Joe Bastianich launched Heritage's first family of accounts and remain our close friends and coconspirators.

I have such great respect for all the restaurant chefs who spend more money per pound to support noncorporate farmers. They are saving our land, our gastronomy, and diversity in our food supply. Please visit our website to see a list of amazing chef/restaurant pioneers — these are the sorts of establishments we should be eating at! Also, thank you to all the forward-thinking home chefs who buy from our mail-order division—you have helped create a food economy that flies in the face of modern trends of culinary mediocrity.

Mario, Teresa, Lou, and Nick Fantasma at Paradise Locker Meats eat even more meat than me, and I have great respect for that. I couldn't do any of this without them and their amazing team. They are the hub of the heritage movement in the USA. Thanks also to Larry Boukal and the team at Cannonball Express for moving it all.

The Heritage Foods USA farmers are the hardest-working people I know. They produce the best food in the world while following the rules of agriculture and God. They are Larry and Madonna Sorrell, Craig and Amy Good, Doug and Betty Metzger, Trent and Troy Baker, Eric Norton, Matt Keevhaver, Joseph Hubbard, Sharon Meyer, Danny Williamson, Dan Flaherty, James and Lisa Twomey, Chris Wilson, Katy and Richard Harjes, Alec Bradford, David and Chris Newman, Jim Davis, Christopher Nicolson, Winona LaDuke, Kevin White, Gina and Brian Batali, Ben Machin, Eric and Callene Rapp, the Schlabach family, Debbie and Steve Farrara, all the goat farmers, Will Harris III, Mr. and Mr. Kenneth, and Long Meadow Ranch.

Thanks to Chris Parachini, Brandon Hoy, and the entire team at Roberta's. A tidal wave of energy flows out of that place each day, and I have learned a tremendous amount from being a part of that amazing community. The radio hosts and team of newswriters are among the most inspiring activists and educators I have ever met. Their work is very important and commands respect.

Special thanks to Caitlin Robin, Ahmed Abushaban, and Aroon Puckpibul, who have each gifted me with an additional thirty minutes of sleep per night through peace of mind!

Sarah Obraitis helped open 80 percent of the wholesale accounts Heritage still has today. Her high energy delivered the idea of "heritage" to the world of food. Todd Wickstrom helped set this Heritage engine in motion and continues to fight for the cause each and every day.

Very special thanks to Carlo Petrini and Alice Waters, Michael Pollan, and all of the first wave of Slow Food USA chapter leaders. Thanks to Steve Jenkins, Ben Flanner, and Billy and Meg for all the beer references. And Marion Nestle for finding us the world's greatest interns at NYU's food studies program.

And Mini Bar and Damon Boelte for feeding us.

Thanks also to Steve Hearst, Rodney Benson, Michael Batterberry, Eric Schlosser, Dave Arnold, Maxine Ganer, FlashTalksCash, Denny Abrams, Peter Izzo, Patrick Fitzsimmons, Rinaldo Frattolillo, Jonathan Russo, Renato Sardo and Angelo Garro, Craig St. John, Al Benton, Nancy Newsome, Armandino Batali, Wes Jackson, Chris Howell, Chris Carpenter, Jeremy Hirsh, Brian Anselmo, EJ DeCoske, Carrie Holland, Andrea Trabucco, John Ruth, Heather Hyman, Dennis O'Conner, Katy Keiffer, Sarah McCoy, Dan Honig,

Julie Shaffer, Michael Piazza, Dan Purdy, Anthony Butler, Mike and Darleen Antocci, Saro di Liberto, Tekserve, Regional Access, Rolling Press, Sara McMonigle, Steve Martocci, Ashley Lawlill, and Bryan and Katie Flannery.

Anne Saxelby proofread countless versions of THE CAR-NIVORE'S MANIFESTO, whether she wanted to or not. She also cowrote the fairy-tale chapter and produced the wonderful drawings that appear throughout the book.

Index

About the Authors

Patrick Martins is an agent of change within the farm and restaurant industry, moving over 60,000 pounds of pasture-raised rare and heritage breeds of pork, beef, and poultry every week from thirty family farms through his company Heritage Foods USA to a client list in ten cities that includes some of America's favorite restaurants and butchers, among them Del Posto, Union Square Cafe, the Spotted Pig, wd~50, Momofuku, Ottomanelli & Sons Meat Market, Morimoto, Oliveto, A16, Quince, Farmstead, Mozza, and more. Heritage Foods USA meats are sourced from breeds that include Red Wattle and Gloucestershire Old Spot pigs, Akaushi and Highland cattle, Bourbon Red and Narragansett turkey, Oberhasli and Kiko goat, and Plymouth Rock and Columbian Wyandotte chicken, which are also sold to home kitchens around the country through their mail order program (www.HeritageFoodsUSA.com).

Prior to launching Heritage Foods USA in 2004, Martins founded Slow Food USA, which he began after he spent a year working in Italy with Slow Food originator, author, and educator Carlo Petrini. Martins is also a founder and an on-air personality of the Heritage Radio Network, which airs daily news coverage on all things food as well as thirty hours of original programming a week. He lives and works in Brooklyn.

Mike Edison is the former editor and publisher of *High Times* magazine and author of the memoir *I Have Fun Everywhere I Go: Savage Tales of Pot, Porn, Punk Rock, Pro Wrestling, Talking Apes, Evil Bosses, Dirty Blues, American Heroes, and the Most Notorious Magazines in the World* (Farrar, Straus & Giroux, 2008). Edison has contributed to numerous magazines and websites, including the *Huffington Post,* the *Daily Beast,* the *New York Observer, Spin,* and the *New York Press,* for whom he covered classical music and professional wrestling. His latest book is *Dirty! Dirty! Dirty!: Of Playboys, Pigs, and Penthouse Paupers; An American Tale of Sex and Wonder* (Soft Skull Press, 2011). More recently he collaborated with Joe Bastianich on his *New York Times* bestselling memoir, *Restaurant Man* (Viking, 2012). Edison is also a well-known musician and storyteller, and performs often with various iterations of his long-running gospel and blues experiment the Edison Rocket Train. He speaks frequently on free speech and the American counterculture, and can also be heard on the Heritage Radio Network on his show *Arts & Seizures.* Edison lives and works in New York City.